The Evolving Landscape of Atopic Dermatitis

Editors

NANETTE B. SILVERBERG
JONATHAN I. SILVERBERG

DERMATOLOGIC CLINICS

www.derm.theclinics.com

Consulting Editor
BRUCE H. THIERS

October 2024 • Volume 42 • Number 4

ELSEVIER

1600 John F. Kennedy Boulevard • Suite 1800 • Philadelphia, Pennsylvania, 19103-2899

http://www.theclinics.com

DERMATOLOGIC CLINICS Volume 42, Number 4
October 2024 ISSN 0733-8635, ISBN-13: 978-0-443-29366-5

Editor: Stacy Eastman
Developmental Editor: Nitesh Barthwal

Dermatologic Clinics (ISSN 0733-8635) is published quarterly by Elsevier Inc., 360 Park Avenue South, New York, NY 10010-1710. Months of publication are January, April, July, and October. Business and editorial offices: 1600 John F. Kennedy Blvd., Suite 1800, Philadelphia, PA 19103-2899. Customer service office: 11830 Westline Drive, St. Louis, MO 63146. Periodicals postage paid at New York, NY, and additional mailing offices. Subscription prices are USD 447.00 per year for US individuals, USD 478.00 per year for Canadian individuals, USD 547.00 per year for international individuals, USD 100.00 per year for US students/residents, USD 100.00 per year for Canadian students/residents, and USD 240 per year for international students/residents. For institutional access pricing please contact Customer Service via the contact information below. International air speed delivery is included in all *Clinics* subscription prices. All prices are subject to change without notice. Orders, claims, and journal inquiries: Please visit our Support Hub page https://service.elsevier.com for assistance.

Reprints. For copies of 100 or more, of articles in this publication, please contact the Commercial Reprints Department, Elsevier Inc., 360 Park Avenue South, New York, New York 10010-1710. Tel.: 212-633-3874; Fax: 212-633-3820; Email: reprints@elsevier.com.

The *Dermatologic Clinics* is covered in *MEDLINE/PubMed (Index Medicus)*, *Current Contents/Clinical Medicine*, *Excerpta Medica*, *Chemical Abstracts*, and *ISI/BIOMED*.

Contributors

CONSULTING EDITOR

BRUCE H. THIERS, MD
Professor and Chairman Emeritus, Department of Dermatology and Dermatologic Surgery,
Medical University of South Carolina, Charleston, South Carolina, USA

EDITORS

NANETTE B. SILVERBERG, MD
Clinical Professor, Departments of Dermatology and Pediatrics, Icahn School of Medicine at Mt. Sinai, New York, New York, USA

JONATHAN I. SILVERBERG, MD, PhD, MPH
Professor, Department of Dermatology, The George Washington University School of Medicine and Health Sciences, Director, Clinical Research and Contact Dermatitis, Washington, DC, USA

AUTHORS

MUDRA BHATT, MBBS
Medical Student, Government Medical College, Bhavnagar, India

SARAH G. BROOKS, BA
Research Fellow, Dr. Phillip Frost Department of Dermatology and Cutaneous Surgery, Miami Itch Center, University of Miami Miller School of Medicine, Coral Gables, Florida, USA

PATRICK M. BRUNNER, MD, MSc
Associate Professor, Department of Dermatology, Icahn School of Medicine at Mount Sinai, New York, New York, USA

MARIA GNARRA BUETHE, MD, PhD
Pediatric Dermatology Fellow, Division of Pediatric and Adolescent Dermatology, Rady Children's Hospital San Diego, San Diego, California, USA; Department of Dermatology, University of California San Diego School of Medicine, La Jolla, California, USA

ZELMA C. CHIESA FUXENCH, MD, MSCE
Assistant Professor, Department of Dermatology, Perelman School of Medicine, University of Pennsylvania, Philadelphia, Pennsylvania, USA

AMANDA COX, MD
Associate Professor of Pediatrics, Division of Pediatric Allergy, Icahn School of Medicine at Mount Sinai, New York, New York, USA

DAVID L. DRUM, BS
Medical Student, California University of Science and Medicine, Colton, California, USA

LAWRENCE F. EICHENFIELD, MD
Distinguished Professor and Chief, Division of Pediatric and Adolescent Dermatology, Rady Children's Hospital San Diego, San Diego, California, USA; Departments of Dermatology and Pediatrics, University of California San Diego School of Medicine, La Jolla, California, USA

WILLIAM FITZMAURICE, BS
Department of Dermatology, Icahn School of Medicine at Mt Sinai, New York, New York, USA

ANIKA G. JALLORINA, BS
Medical Student, California University of Science and Medicine, Colton, California, USA

JESSICA K. JOHNSON, MPH
Director of Community Research and
Engagement, National Eczema Association,
Novato, California, USA

CAITLYN KELLOGG, MD
Associate Physician, Division of Pediatric and
Adolescent Dermatology, Rady Children's
Hospital San Diego, San Diego, California,
USA; Department of Dermatology, University of
California San Diego School of Medicine, La
Jolla, California, USA

KARAN LAL, DO, MS
Dermatologist, Affiliated Dermatology,
Scottsdale, Arizona, USA; Department of
Dermatology, Northwell Health, Glen Cove,
New York, USA

MARY F. LEE-WONG, MD, MS, MSc
Chief, Division of Adult Allergy and
Immunology, Maimonides Medical Center,
Brooklyn, New York, USA; Professor Emeritus,
Division of Allergy and Immunology,
Department of Medicine, Icahn School of
Medicine at Mount Sinai, New York, New York,
USA

SHANTHI NARLA, MD
Assistant Professor, Department of
Dermatology, Medical College of Wisconsin,
Milwaukee, Wisconsin, USA

LAUREN R. PORT, BA
Medical Student, Department of Dermatology,
Icahn School of Medicine at Mount Sinai, New
York, New York, USA

KEVIN PUERTA DURANGO, BS
Research Fellow, Department of Dermatology,
Perelman School of Medicine, University of
Pennsylvania, Philadelphia, Pennsylvania, USA

MYKAYLA SANDLER, BA
Research Fellow, Department of Dermatology,
Massachusetts General Hospital, Medical
Student, Harvard Medical School, Boston,
Massachusetts, USA

YOUNG JOON SEO, MD
Professor, Division of Pediatric and Adolescent
Dermatology, Rady Children's Hospital San
Diego, San Diego, California, USA; Department

of Dermatology, University of California San
Diego School of Medicine, La Jolla, California,
USA; Department of Dermatology, Chungnam
National University College of Medicine,
Daejeon, Korea

AMI SHAH, MD
Physician, Division of Allergy and Immunology,
Icahn School of Medicine at Mount Sinai, New
York, New York, USA

SCOTT H. SICHERER, MD
Director, Professor of Pediatric Allergy and
Immunology, Division of Allergy and
Immunology, Professor of Pediatrics, Division
of Pediatric Allergy, Icahn School of Medicine
at Mount Sinai, New York, New York, USA

JONATHAN I. SILVERBERG, MD, PhD, MPH
Professor, Department of Dermatology, The
George Washington University School of
Medicine and Health Sciences, Director,
Clinical Research and Contact Dermatitis,
Washington, DC, USA

NANETTE B. SILVERBERG, MD
Clinical Professor, Departments of
Dermatology and Pediatrics, Icahn School of
Medicine at Mt. Sinai, New York, New York,
USA

WENDY SMITH BEGOLKA, MBS
Chief Strategy Officer, Research Medical, and
Community Affairs, National Eczema
Association, Novato, California, USA

ISABELLE J. THIBAU, MPH
Director of EczemaWise Growth and
Implementation, National Eczema Association,
Novato, California, USA

BRIT TROGEN, MD, MS
Allergy Immunology Fellow, Division of
Pediatric Allergy, Icahn School of Medicine at
Mount Sinai, New York, New York, USA

ANGELA TSUANG, MD, MSc
Assistant Professor, Division of Allergy and
Immunology, Icahn School of Medicine at
Mount Sinai, New York, New York, USA

MEGHA VERMA, DO
Internal Medical Resident, Department of
Internal Medicine, Mount Sinai Morningside/
West, New York, New York, USA

CARRIE VUONG, MD
Dermatologist, Division of Pediatric and
Adolescent Dermatology, Rady Children's
Hospital San Diego, San Diego, California,
USA; Department of Dermatology, University of
California San Diego School of Medicine, La
Jolla, California, USA

LEO S. WAN, BA
Medical Student, West Virginia School of
Osteopathic Medicine, Lewisburg, West
Virginia, USA

GIL YOSIPOVITCH, MD
Professor, Dr. Phillip Frost Department of
Dermatology and Cutaneous Surgery,
Miami Itch Center, University of Miami Miller
School of Medicine, Coral Gables, Florida,
USA

JIADE YU, MD, MS
Assistant Professor, Department of
Dermatology, Massachusetts General
Hospital, Harvard Medical School, Boston,
Massachusetts, USA

Contents

The longitudinal course of atopic dermatitis (AD) is heterogeneous and complex. While previously thought to be a childhood disorder, recent studies demonstrated that childhood-onset AD may take several different courses that may involve persistence into adulthood becoming a lifelong condition. Other patients only demonstrated adult-onset AD. Different factors may play a role in the timing of AD onset. Assessing the longitudinal course also involves understanding the changing temporal pattern of AD. Understanding the dynamic course of AD is important in identifying individualized treatment recommendations for patients.

Atopic Dermatitis (AD) is a common, pruritic inflammatory skin disease associated with marked disease burden and substantial health care costs. AD does not discriminate between populations; prevalence estimates vary widely with most studies focusing on general or pediatric populations and a limited number of studies in adult populations solely. The costs of treating AD are staggering. Studies that examine differences in prevalence may be difficult to compare due to differences in study designs. However, understanding the prevalence of AD across populations is critical if we are to improve the lives of patients and caregivers living with this disease.

Atopic dermatitis (AD) and food allergies are 2 atopic conditions that tend to develop early in life. Their interrelationship has been a topic of controversy and many studies. The presence of atopic dermatitis in infancy and early childhood, particularly if severe, is a risk factor for the development of immunoglobulin E (IgE) -mediated food allergies. While it is common for children with AD to demonstrate extensive sensitization to foods, serum IgE testing is not always indicative of clinical allergy.

Atopic dermatitis (AD) is a complex, chronic disease with multiple negative impacts to patients' health, lives, and overall well-being. The lived experience of AD is multi-dimensional, heterogeneous, and ever-changing, yet an essential contributor to a holistic understanding of disease burden. Real-world self-monitoring of disease burden by patients has potential as a valuable adjunct to clinical and patient-reported assessments in health care settings. Newer digital tools are available to support

these activities, providing opportunity for patients and health care providers to identify aspects of self-monitoring that can best support AD care and management
goals, treatment outcomes, and minimize patient burden.

Atopic dermatitis is an inflammatory skin condition that largely affects children.
Atopic dermatitis has the potential to persist into adulthood and continue to negatively affect the lives of those who are burdened with it. This condition can have a
large impact on the quality of life of those who are affected from birth through senescence. Scoring systems have been developed over time to help assess the impact
that AD has on an individual's quality of life. The goal of this article is to create an
overview of the quality of life scores by age group and across nationalities.

Patients with atopic dermatitis (AD) are at increased risk of atopic and non-atopic
comorbidities. In fact, the Hanifin and Rajka criteria include allergic and infectious
comorbidities as a minor criterion. Despite the well-recognized list of comorbidities,
the past 15 years greatly expanded the list of recognized comorbidities of AD. This
narrative review focuses on comorbidities of AD using a mnemonic, VINDICATE-P:
vascular/cardiovascular, infectious, neoplastic and neurologic, degenerative, iatrogenic, congenital, atopic and autoimmune, traumatic, endocrine/metabolic, and
psychiatric. The comorbidities of AD vary by age. More research is needed into
the mechanisms of comorbidities and optimal screening strategies in AD patients.

Atopic dermatitis (AD) is a chronic inflammatory skin disorder that requires a complex management strategy, which often involves multiple and diverse topicals and
systemic treatment regimens. While topical steroids and more recently calcineurin
inhibitors have been the mainstay therapy for mild-to-moderate disease, recent advances in the understanding of AD pathogenesis have led to the development of different new targets, rapidly widening our therapeutic armamentarium. This review
summarizes their efficacy and safety data. We also review topical optimization strategies, including the recently published topical volume calculator, to maximize long-
term disease control, especially when using multiple agents at the same time.

Atopic dermatitis (AD) is a chronic inflammatory skin condition that can be difficult to
treat due to a complex etiology and diverse clinical presentations. Itch is the most
common symptom associated with AD with profound negative impact on quality
of life. Thus, the adjunctive management of itch in patients with AD is needed to control and reduce disease burden. Supplemental treatment options are continuously
emerging and undergoing testing in clinical trials. This article summarizes the latest

data on topical and systemic adjunctive therapies for AD safety and efficacy in reducing itch.

Ami Shah, Scott H. Sicherer, and Angela Tsuang

Recommendations about allergy prevention through diet are rapidly changing. In just the past several years, multiple organizations have provided updated guidance and recommendations about infant feeding based on recent studies and meta-analyses. In addition to the increased number of studies supporting the benefit of early introduction of allergenic foods, in particular peanut and egg, recent studies demonstrate that infant and maternal diet diversity may also reduce risk of food allergy and atopy. Skin emollients have not been found to be helpful in prevention of food allergy, and more evidence is needed to determine if emollients play a role in prevention of atopic dermatitis.

Mykayla Sandler and JiaDe Yu

Atopic dermatitis (AD) and allergic contact dermatitis (ACD) are common inflammatory skin diseases in both children and adults that present similarly and often coexist. Patch testing is the gold standard for establishing the diagnosis of ACD and can often help distinct between the 2 conditions. Patch testing is more challenging in patients with underlying AD due to potential for angry back reactions. In this review, we discuss the current evidence and guidelines regarding the screening for contact allergies in patients with AD. We also discuss the most frequent relevant allergens in adults and children with atopic dermatitis.

Mudra Bhatt, Karan Lal, and Nanette B. Silverberg

Atopic dermatitis (AD) begins in early childhood in the majority of children. Addressing AD in small children includes recognition of the early presentations of disease in all skin types, triggers, comorbidities, and therapeutics. These include risk of medication absorption, more xerosis, infections, and creating management plans that are acceptable to parents/caregivers, while offering safety. Vaccination efficacy, safety on systemic agents, growth and development, tactile sensory development, and teething-related facial eruptions of early childhood are additional concerns. Prevention of long-term comorbidities is the highest goal. Using age-based considerations helps support excellence in care and improved patient–parent experience.

Lauren R. Port and Patrick M. Brunner

Atopic hand dermatitis (AHD), a manifestation of atopic dermatitis, can have a profound negative effect on a patient's disease-related quality of life due to its visibility, chronic nature, and overall discomfort that it causes. AHD differs from other forms of chronic hand eczema due to its likely distinct, complex pathogenesis, which is a combination of environmental triggers, genetic predisposition, and immune dysfunction. A proper diagnosis of AHD is made through clinical evaluation and the ability to establish subtle clinical differences between AHD and other conditions.

DERMATOLOGIC CLINICS

SERIES OF RELATED INTEREST

Medical Clinics
https://www.medical.theclinics.com/
Immunology and Allergy Clinics
https://www.immunology.theclinics.com/
Clinics in Plastic Surgery
https://www.plasticsurgery.theclinics.com/
Otolaryngologic Clinics
https://www.oto.theclinics.com/

Preface

Atopic Dermatitis: The Era of Excellence in Care

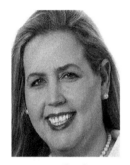

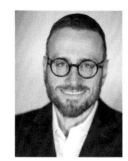

Nanette B. Silverberg, MD   Jonathan I. Silverberg, MD, PhD, MPH

Editors

Atopic dermatitis (AD) is a chronic inflammatory skin and multisystem disorder characterized by atopy in the patients and family members. AD affects patients from shortly after birth through senescence, and this lifetime of disease is accompanied by altered morphologies with time, differences in needs, and in particular, quality-of-life impairment. In this issue, the best clinicians in dermatology, pediatric dermatology, allergy, and immunology provide insight into management strategies they use to provide excellence in care, a combination of prevention of disease and comorbidity onset and severity, disease and symptom control, prevention of flares, and patient satisfaction.

One can only understand AD through the lens of the global burden of AD. Durango and colleagues highlight the worldwide burden that has grown in the past 50 years and remains an unremitting trend.

It is a common misunderstanding by patients and caregivers to believe foods are the origin of AD. Despite the misunderstanding, the comorbidity of food allergy is incredibly significant in that it can confer long-term disease severity, and if left unchecked, creates a potential nidus for AD flare and potentially worse, for example, anaphylaxis. Shah and colleagues highlight advances in the timing of food introduction and allergy prevention. Their article distills decades of novel interventions and advancements in the prevention and mitigation

of patients suffering with food allergy. Trogen and colleagues bring this issue home by highlighting the role of food allergy in AD. The pair of articles identifies the on-going need for dermatologists and allergists to maintain open discourse in order to provide our patients with maximal care.

AD is a lifetime disease; therefore, consideration for management strategies must address all age groups to produce excellence. Narla and colleagues look at the long-term course of AD, addressing the lifespan. Bhatt and colleagues address special considerations for younger children, identifying management strategies pertinent to the younger child.

Burden of disease is a key element in understanding patient symptoms and promoting patient satisfaction. Begolka and colleagues discuss burden from the patient perspective, including patient self-monitoring strategies. Their points highlight the patient voice. Fitzmaurice and colleagues address the long-term impact of AD on quality of life, highlighting the need for a variety of instruments to obtain long- and short-term perspectives on quality-of-life impairment.

Creating the healthiest and most symptom-free AD patient is an essential goal of AD care, as we promote excellence in disease control and outcomes. Excellence in AD care includes addressing important comorbidities. In this issue, the comorbidities of AD are abbreviated as a new mnemonic,

Dermatol Clin 42 (2024) xiii–xiv
https://doi.org/10.1016/j.det.2024.07.001
0733-8635/24/© 2024 Published by Elsevier Inc.

VINDICATE-P. Considering disease comorbidities as preventable highlights how prevention of food allergy remains a linked entity to AD excellence in care. Sandler and colleagues highlight how comanagement of allergic contact dermatitis in AD promotes best outcomes in care. Brunner and colleagues further highlight the importance of hand dermatitis as a manifestation of AD. Drum and colleagues provide an overview of emerging data on the linkage of AD with cancers, highlighting how aberrant skin immunity can link the skin to cancer in virtually any organ.

Excellence in care requires therapeutic interventions to control disease, reducing disease activity and flaring. Buethe and colleagues highlight the latest approaches to excellence in skin-directed topical management. Griffiths Brooks and colleagues address best practices to control itch in AD, a symptom that is so frequently reduced, but so rarely eliminated.

This medley of articles from epidemiologic to therapeutic highlights the richness of AD research and the multitude of approaches that harmonize to produce disease clearance and long-term control, that is, excellence in care.

DISCLOSURES

N.B. Silverberg has been an investigator for Avita and a speaker or consultant for Regeneron, Incyte, Verrica, Novan, Apogee, Loreal, and Primus Pharmaceuticals. J.I. Silverberg has received honoraria as a consultant and/or advisory board member for Abbvie, Alamar, Aldena, Amgen, AObiome, Apollo, Arcutis, Arena, Asana, Aslan, Attovia, BioMX, Biosion, Bodewell, Boehringer-Ingelheim, Bristell-Meyers Squibb, Cara, Castle Biosciences, Celgene, Connect Biopharma, Corevitas, Dermavant, Eli Lilly, FIDE, Galderma, GlaxoSmithKline, Incyte, Inmagene, Invea, Kiniksa, Leo Pharma, Merck, My-Or Diagnostics, Nektar, Novartis, Optum, Pfizer, RAPT, Recludix, Regeneron, Sandoz, Sanofi-Genzyme, Shaperon, TARGET-RWE, Teva, Union, UpToDate; speaker for Abbvie, Eli Lilly, Leo Pharma, Pfizer, Regeneron, Sanofi-Genzyme.

Nanette B. Silverberg, MD
Departments of Dermatology and Pediatrics
Icahn School of Medicine at Mt. Sinai
5 E 98th Street
New York, NY 10029, USA

Jonathan I. Silverberg, MD, PhD, MPH
Department of Dermatology
The George Washington University
School of Medicine and Health Sciences
Suite 2B-430
2150 Pennsylvania Avenue
Washington, DC 20037, USA

E-mail addresses:
Nanette.silverberg@mountsinai.org
(N.B. Silverberg)
JonathanISilverberg@gmail.com (J.I. Silverberg)

Atopic Dermatitis
A Disorder of both Adults and Children with Varying Longitudinal Course

Shanthi Narla, MD[a], Jonathan I. Silverberg, MD, PhD, MPH[b],*

KEYWORDS

• Atopic dermatitis • Longitudinal course • Age-of-onset • Temporal patterns • Aging

KEY POINTS

• Atopic dermatitis (AD) is more common in adults than previously thought, and it encompasses persistent childhood AD as well as adult-onset AD.
• An important part of understanding the longitudinal course of AD involves recognizing the changing temporal pattern, including fluctuation, persistence, and improvement.
• Only considering health care assessments at the time of visit may not be sufficient enough to assess the longitudinal course of AD.
• Each combination of AD severity and persistence has its own specific treatment considerations.

INTRODUCTION

Atopic dermatitis (AD) is common in both children and adults and has a variable longitudinal course. The prevalence of AD in the United States was approximately 13% among children and 7% among adults.[1–5] In the United Kingdom, active AD affected 12.3% of children aged 0 to 17 years, 5.1% of adults aged 18 to 74 years, and 8.7% of adults aged 75 to 99 years.[6] Prevalent cases of AD in adults may be due to persistent childhood AD or adult-onset AD.[1]

Patients and parents of children with AD often ask, "Can my child 'grow out' of eczema?" or "I never had eczema as a kid, can you get it as an adult?" This narrative review will summarize the most recent data regarding the longitudinal course of AD in children and adults and will address the differences in AD presentation in different ages of onset. Understanding the disease course is important to identifying appropriate treatment interventions.

AGE OF ONSET

AD can start at any age. Approximately 60% to 73% of children with AD reportedly have disease onset before 1 to 2 years of age.[7–9] A systematic review (SR) of 25 studies including patients aged 16 years or older found that approximately 1 in 4 adults with AD reported adult-onset disease (range: 10%–60%), with higher proportions of adult-onset disease reported among studies with longer durations of follow-up.[10–12]

Many age-related skin changes occur that may contribute to the development of adult-onset AD. For example, skin-barrier function diminishes, including downregulation of filaggrin, claudin-1 and occludin proteins, and decreased barrier repair after irritation.[13–16] Filaggrin null mutations are a strong genetic risk factor particularly for childhood-onset AD. AD is also characterized by reduced expression of claudin-1 and claudin-23 in adult and increased transepidermal water loss in both adult and child nonlesional AD skin.[15,17–20]

---

[a] Department of Dermatology, Medical College of Wisconsin, Office A3698, 8701 Watertown Plank Road, Milwaukee, WI 53226, USA; [b] Department of Dermatology, The George Washington University School of Medicine and Health Sciences, Suite 2B-430, 2150 Pennsylvania Avenue, Washington, DC 20037, USA
* Corresponding author.
E-mail address: JonathanISilverberg@Gmail.com

Dermatol Clin 42 (2024) 513–518
https://doi.org/10.1016/j.det.2024.05.002
0733-8635/24/© 2024 Elsevier Inc. All rights reserved.

Both age-related skin changes and AD are characterized by diminished function of pattern recognition receptors and phagocytic function of polymorphonuclear leukocytes (ie, dysregulation of the innate immune system).[15,21–24] As the skin ages, adaptive immunity may also shift toward Th2 processes.[25] Immunoglobulin E (IgE)+ CD1a+ dendritic cells and mast cells are increased in the aging skin, as well as an increased risk of *Staphylococcus aureus* infections in patients aged 65 years or older.[15,26–30] Studies demonstrate higher rates of *S aureus* infections early in life, a low incidence through young adulthood, and a gradual rise in incidence with advancing age.[15,26–32]

A German study of 834 women found that exposures to nitrogen oxides and particulate matter were associated with an increased incidence of eczema, particularly nonatopic eczema.[33] Associations with air pollution were stronger in carriers of fewer risk alleles for atopic eczema.[33] This suggests that eczema in the elderly may differ from genetically driven atopic eczema. Environmental factors, such as air pollution and skin barrier function, may be more relevant to the development of eczema in the elderly population, especially for nonatopic type of eczema, and the atopic diathesis may be less important for the development of eczema in the elderly.[33] Another study found that current and ever smoking, and number of packs per year were risk factors for adult-onset AD, as well as environmental exposure to tobacco smoke among nonsmokers.[34]

LONGITUDINAL COURSE OF ATOPIC DERMATITIS
In Children

Several studies examined the course of childhood AD over time.[35–38] A study of children and adolescents in the United Kingdom and Netherlands identified 6 different disease trajectories: early-onset-persistent, early-onset-late resolving, early-onset-early resolving, mid-onset-resolving, late-onset-resolving, and unaffected/transient.[37] In a Singaporean cohort, early-onset transient, late-onset persistent, and early-onset persistent were identified as childhood AD trajectories.[36] Another study identified 4 different eczema phenotypes: early-transient, mid-transient, late transient, and persistent eczema.[38] Patients may benefit from tailored treatment to these various disease courses; however, there may also be significant overlap between the disease trajectories.

Some controversy remains about how commonly childhood AD persists into adulthood and estimates of persistence vary widely across studies. A longitudinal study of 7157 children from the Pediatric Eczema Elective Registry (PEER) cohort found that at every age (2–26 years), more than 80% of patients had AD symptoms and/or were using medication to treat their AD. It was not until age 20 years that 50% of patients experienced a 6 month period that was symptom and treatment free, further suggesting that AD is likely a life-long condition.[39] A subsequent study from the PEER cohort found that history of atopy (including food and animal allergies), female sex, annual family income of less than US$50,000 at enrollment, non-White race, and younger age at eczema onset, and frequent use of AD medications at a younger age were predictors of persistently active AD.[40] In longitudinal analyses, older AD onset age was associated with better control and less persistence (early-onset ≤2 years vs mid-onset 3–7 years, late-onset 8–17 years).[41] However, a limitation of the PEER cohort is that only a select group of patients with chronic persistent AD using a topical calcineurin inhibitor were enrolled.

An SR and meta-analysis of 7 longitudinal studies (n = 13,515) found the decrease in prevalence after the age of 12 years was 1%, which was not statistically significant. Similar results were found with other age cutoffs.[42] These results suggest that the reason for steady prevalence estimates across ages could be due to a combination of active disease in both childhood and early adulthood among some individuals, remission or clearance of disease among others, and late-onset disease among others.[42] In a prospective cohort study of eighth grade children in 1995 followed until 2010, the persistence of AD in childhood was common and significantly affected quality of life. Persistent AD was particularly prevalent in those with early-onset, allergic rhinitis, and hand eczema.[43]

In contrast, an SR and meta-analysis of 45 studies from 15 different countries found that 80% of childhood AD did not persist by 8 years of age and less than 5% persisted by 20 years after diagnosis, and children who developed AD by the age of 2 years had less persistence.[44] The mean duration of AD persistence was 3.0 years.[44] Persistence was greater in studies using patient/caregiver-assessed versus physician-assessed outcomes, those with more severe AD, in female individuals versus male individuals, but not in those with sensitivity to allergens (positive skin-prick testing and/or antigen-specific serum IgE).[44] Persistence was defined as the presence of AD on consecutive study visits.[44] This definition does not capture the occurrence of subsequent AD flares and likely underestimates the proportion of individuals who continue to experience disease activity. Nevertheless, these results suggest that early-onset AD does tend to "burn out" and improve by adulthood. However, children with later onset, more persistent AD, and severe AD may be much more likely to have prolonged persistence into adolescence and adulthood.[44] The associated higher persistence of AD reported in patient/caregiver assessments versus physician assessments may further reflect the varied course of AD, emphasizing that patient-reported outcomes are just as important as physician-reported outcomes in determining severity. These risk factors may be useful to predict which children will have persistent AD.[44]

Few studies examined the role of race or ethnicity on childhood AD persistence. In a prospective cohort study of 4898 women and their children born in 20 large US cities between 1998 and 2000, prevalence was determined at ages 5, 9, and 15 years. The results found that female sex and Black race were associated with persistent AD across all 3 ages.[45] In a prospective pre-birth cohort in eastern Massachusetts, using multivariable logistic regression adjusting for sociodemographic factors, non-Hispanic Blacks and Hispanics with early childhood AD were more likely to have persistent AD.[46] In an African-American cohort with AD, Filaggrin 2 mutations were associated with more persistent AD.[47]

In Adults

Less is known about the longitudinal course of AD in adults. A prospective US dermatology-practice based study of 400 adult patients with AD found that 36.2% had moderate and 18.2% had severe Eczema Area and Severity Index (EASI) scores at any visit over a 2 year observation period; 29.0% had moderate and 26.4% had severe objective-SCORing Atopic Dermatitis (SCORAD) scores at any visit. Among patients with baseline moderate or severe EASI scores, 25.0% and 18.6% continued to have moderate or severe scores at 1 or more follow-up visits, respectively. Among patients with baseline moderate or severe objective-SCORAD scores, 22.6% and 24.5% continued to have moderate or severe scores at 1 or more follow-up visits, respectively.[48] Similarly, in the International Study of Life with Atopic Eczema (that consisted of 2002 patients and caregivers from 8 countries, with >60% of the patients being >13 years of age), patients experienced on an average 9 flares per year, lasting 15 days at a time. In total, patients spent 136 days per year in AD flare. Patients with severe disease experienced more frequent (11.1 per year) and longer (173 days) flares than the total sample.[49]

CLINICAL RELEVANCE OF LONGITUDINAL COURSE

An important part of understanding the longitudinal course of AD involves recognizing its variable temporal patterns, including fluctuation, persistence, and resolution. Only considering cross-sectional health care assessments at the time of visit does not sufficiently characterize the longitudinal course. For example, a patient may have been flaring and hospitalized 2 weeks earlier but have clear skin during the encounter.

Several AD phenotypes may exist: (1) good control, (2) seasonally moderate–severe, (3) frequent moderate flares, (4) moderate with severe flares, and (5) chronic severe. Good control is characterized by stability over time with transient mild worsening of AD with no major disease fluctuation.[50] These patients can be optimized with intermittent use of topical anti-inflammatory agents and gentle skin care.[50] Seasonally moderate–severe AD is characterized by 1 or 2 major flares per year in a particular season or with change of seasons but is otherwise well controlled.[50] This course of AD may benefit from short-term topical or systemic treatments with rapid-onset strong efficacy that can be used intermittently, for example, topical corticosteroids or Janus kinase (JAK) inhibitors, oral corticosteroids, cyclosporine, or oral JAK inhibitors (off-label use).[50] Multiple courses of topical or lower dose systemic oral immunomodulators may be needed to treat frequent, moderate flares, and chronic treatment with biologic, phototherapy, or lower dose oral systemic immunomodulators may be needed to prevent the flares and achieve long-term disease control.[50] Continuous therapy with a biologic may be the best course of action for patients with baseline moderate AD with severe flares. Finally, patients with chronic severe AD may require a combination of treatment modalities, for example, oral JAK inhibitors, biologics, and/or phototherapy.[50]

Each combination of AD severity and persistence has its own specific treatment considerations. For example, flares require treatments with quick onset and strong efficacy. Maintenance agents need to be used safely in the long term for flare prevention. The heterogeneous temporal pattern of AD should be incorporated into clinical practice to better set realistic expectations for patients.

SUMMARY

It is important for clinicians to recognize the heterogeneous clinical course of AD in different age groups. While traditionally thought of as a childhood disorder, increasing evidence suggests persistence of AD into adulthood, and adult-onset AD is very common. The heterogeneous course of AD should be addressed when selecting AD treatments.

CLINICS CARE POINTS

- There are conflicting studies on how often childhood AD persists into adulthood.

- Later childhood onset, already persistent AD, and greater AD severity may be associated with increased persistence of childhood AD into adulthood.

- Environmental factors, such as air pollution, and skin barrier function may be more relevant to the development of eczema in the elderly population, especially for nonatopic type of eczema, and the atopic diathesis may be less important for the development of eczema in the elderly.

- Cross-sectional health care assessments may not accurately characterize a patient's longitudinal course of AD. Patient/caregiver-reported assessments also need to be considered to gain a thorough understanding of the patient's severity and course.

AUTHOR CONTRIBUTIONS

Drafting of the article: S. Narla and J.I. Silverberg; critical revision of the article for important intellectual content: S. Narla and J.I. Silverberg; administrative technical or material support: None; study supervision: None.

DISCLOSURE

S. Narla is a subinvestigator for Janssen, Takeda, and Eli Lilly. J.I. Silverberg has received honoraria as a consultant and/or advisory board member for AbbVie, Afyx, Arena, Asana, BioMX, Bluefin, Bodewell, Boehringer-Ingelheim, Celgene, Dermavant, Dermira, Eli Lilly, Galderma, GlaxoSmithKline, Incyte, Kiniksa, Leo, Luna, Menlo, Novartis, Pfizer, RAPT, Regeneron, and Sanofi; data safety monitoring committee member for Afyx, Hoth, and Morphosys; speaker for Pfizer, Regeneron, and Sanofi-Genzyme; institution received grants from Galderma, Switzerland. Funding support: Not applicable. Ethics approval: Not applicable. Consent to participate: Not applicable. Availability of data and material: Not applicable. Code availability: Not applicable.

REFERENCES

1. Silverberg JI. Public Health Burden and Epidemiology of Atopic Dermatitis. Dermatol Clin 2017; 35(3):283–9.

2. Hua T, Silverberg JI. Atopic dermatitis in US Adults: Epidemiology, association with marital status, and atopy. Ann Allergy Asthma Immunol : official publication of the American College of Allergy, Asthma, & Immunology 2018;121(5):622–4.

3. Chiesa Fuxench ZC, Block JK, Boguniewicz M, et al. Atopic Dermatitis in America Study: A Cross-Sectional Study Examining the Prevalence and Disease Burden of Atopic Dermatitis in the US adult Population. J Invest Dermatol 2019;139(3):583–90.

4. Silverberg JI, Gelfand JM, Margolis DJ, et al. Atopic Dermatitis in US Adults: From Population to Health Care Utilization. J Allergy Clin Immunol Pract 2019; 7(5):1524–32.e1522.

5. Silverberg JI, Simpson EL. Associations of childhood eczema severity: a US population-based study. Dermatitis : contact, atopic, occupational, drug 2014;25(3):107–14.

6. Prevalence of Atopic Eczema Among Patients Seen in Primary Care: Data From The Health Improvement Network. Ann Intern Med 2019;170(5):354–6.

7. Kay J, Gawkrodger DJ, Mortimer MJ, et al. The prevalence of childhood atopic eczema in a general population. J Am Acad Dermatol 1994;30(1):35–9.

8. Weidinger S, Novak N. Atopic dermatitis. Lancet (London, England) 2016;387(10023):1109–22.

9. Wan J, Mitra N, Hoffstad OJ, et al. Variations in risk of asthma and seasonal allergies between early- and late-onset pediatric atopic dermatitis: A cohort study. J Am Acad Dermatol 2017;77(4):634–40.

10. Lee HH, Patel KR, Singam V, et al. A systematic review and meta-analysis of the prevalence and phenotype of adult-onset atopic dermatitis. J Am Acad Dermatol 2019;80(6):1526–32.e1527.

11. Salava A, Rieppo R, Lauerma A, et al. Age-dependent Distribution of Atopic Dermatitis in Primary Care: A Nationwide Population-based Study from Finland. Acta Derm Venereol 2022;102:adv00738.

12. Abuabara K, Ye M, McCulloch CE, et al. Clinical onset of atopic eczema: Results from 2 nationally representative British birth cohorts followed through midlife. J Allergy Clin Immunol 2019;144(3):710–9.

13. Rinnerthaler M, Duschl J, Steinbacher P, et al. Age-related changes in the composition of the cornified envelope in human skin. Exp Dermatol 2013;22(5): 329–35.

14. Jin SP, Han SB, Kim YK, et al. Changes in tight junction protein expression in intrinsic aging and photo-aging in human skin in vivo. J Dermatol Sci 2016; 84(1):99–101.

15. Williamson S, Merritt J, De Benedetto A. Atopic dermatitis in the elderly: a review of clinical and

pathophysiological hallmarks. Br J Dermatol 2020; 182(1):47–54.

16. Ghadially R, Brown BE, Sequeira-Martin SM, et al. The aged epidermal permeability barrier. Structural, functional, and lipid biochemical abnormalities in humans and a senescent murine model. J Clin Invest 1995;95(5):2281–90.

17. De Benedetto A, Rafaels NM, McGirt LY, et al. Tight junction defects in patients with atopic dermatitis. J Allergy Clin Immunol 2011;127(3):773–86. e771-777.

18. Gupta J, Grube E, Lucky A, et al. Transepidermal Water Loss As A Biological Marker In Atopic Dermatitis In Children. J Allergy Clin Immunol 2007;119(1): S280.

19. Janssens M, van Smeden J, Gooris GS, et al. Increase in short-chain ceramides correlates with an altered lipid organization and decreased barrier function in atopic eczema patients. J Lipid Res 2012;53(12):2755–66.

20. Toncic R, Kezic S, Jakasa I, et al. Filaggrin Loss-of-function Mutations and levels of Filaggrin Degradation products in adult Patients with Atopic Dermatitis in Croatia. J Eur Acad Dermatol Venereolad 2020; 34(8):1789–94.

21. Shaw AC, Goldstein DR, Montgomery RR. Age-dependent dysregulation of innate immunity. Nat Rev Immunol 2013;13(12):875–87.

22. Kollmann TR, Levy O, Montgomery RR, et al. Innate immune function by Toll-like receptors: distinct responses in newborns and the elderly. Immunity 2012;37(5):771–83.

23. Montgomery RR, Shaw AC. Paradoxical changes in innate immunity in aging: recent progress and new directions. J Leukoc Biol 2015;98(6):937–43.

24. McGirt LY, Beck LA. Innate immune defects in atopic dermatitis. J Allergy Clin Immunol 2006;118(1): 202–8.

25. Hakim FT, Gress RE. Immunosenescence: deficits in adaptive immunity in the elderly. Tissue Antigens 2007;70(3):179–89.

26. Tun K, Shurko JF, Ryan L, et al. Age-based health and economic burden of skin and soft tissue infections in the United States, 2000 and 2012. PLoS One 2018;13(11):e0206893.

27. Laupland KB, Lyytikäinen O, Sgaard M, et al. The changing epidemiology of Staphylococcus aureus bloodstream infection: a multinational population-based surveillance study. Clin Microbiol Infection 2013;19(5):465–71.

28. Yoshikawa TT, Bradley SF. Staphylococcus aureus Infections and Antibiotic Resistance in Older Adults. Clin Infect Dis 2002;34(2):211–6.

29. Thorlacius-Ussing L, Sandholdt H, Larsen AR, et al. Age-Dependent Increase in Incidence of Staphylococcus aureus Bacteremia, Denmark, 2008-2015. Emerg Infect Dis 2019;25(5):875–82.

30. El Atrouni WI, Knoll BM, Lahr BD, et al. Temporal Trends in the Incidence of Staphylococcus aureus Bacteremia in Olmsted County, Minnesota, 1998 to 2005: A Population-Based Study. Clin Infect Dis 2009;49(12):e130–8.

31. Cassat JE, Thomsen I. Staphylococcus aureus infections in children. Curr Opin Infect Dis 2021; 34(5):510–8.

32. Carroll KC, Gadala A, Milstone AM, et al. Trends in pediatric community-onset Staphylococcus aureus antibiotic susceptibilities over a five-year period in a multihospital health system. Antimicrobial Stewardship & Healthcare Epidemiology 2023;3(1): e12.

33. Hüls A, Abramson MJ, Sugiri D, et al. Nonatopic eczema in elderly women: Effect of air pollution and genes. J Allergy Clin Immunol 2019;143(1): 378–85.e379.

34. Lee CH, Chuang HY, Hong CH, et al. Lifetime exposure to cigarette smoking and the development of adult-onset atopic dermatitis. Br J Dermatol 2011; 164(3):483–9.

35. Roduit C, Frei R, Depner M, et al. Phenotypes of Atopic Dermatitis Depending on the Timing of Onset and Progression in Childhood. JAMA Pediatr 2017; 171(7):655–62.

36. Suaini NHA, Yap GC, Bui DPT, et al. Atopic dermatitis trajectories to age 8 years in the GUSTO cohort. Clin Exp Allergy 2021;51(9):1195–206.

37. Paternoster L, Savenije OEM, Heron J, et al. Identification of atopic dermatitis subgroups in children from 2 longitudinal birth cohorts. J Allergy Clin Immunol 2018;141(3):964–71.

38. Hu C, Duijts L, Erler NS, et al. Most associations of early-life environmental exposures and genetic risk factors poorly differentiate between eczema phenotypes: the Generation R Study. Br J Dermatol 2019; 181(6):1190–7.

39. Margolis JS, Abuabara K, Bilker W, et al. Persistence of mild to moderate atopic dermatitis. JAMA Dermatol 2014;150(6):593–600.

40. Abuabara K, Hoffstad O, Troxel AB, et al. Patterns and predictors of atopic dermatitis disease control past childhood: An observational cohort study. J Allergy Clin Immunol 2018;141(2):778–80.e776.

41. Wan J, Mitra N, Hoffstad OJ, et al. Longitudinal atopic dermatitis control and persistence vary with timing of disease onset in children: A cohort study. J Am Acad Dermatol 2019;81(6):1292–9.

42. Abuabara K, Yu AM, Okhovat JP, et al. The prevalence of atopic dermatitis beyond childhood: A systematic review and meta-analysis of longitudinal studies. Allergy 2018;73(3):696–704.

43. Mortz CG, Andersen KE, Dellgren C, et al. Atopic dermatitis from adolescence to adulthood in the TOACS cohort: prevalence, persistence and comorbidities. Allergy 2015;70(7):836–45.

44. Kim JP, Chao LX, Simpson EL, et al. Persistence of atopic dermatitis (AD): A systematic review and meta-analysis. J Am Acad Dermatol 2016;75(4): 681–7.e611.

45. McKenzie C, Silverberg JI. The prevalence and persistence of atopic dermatitis in urban United States children. Ann Allergy Asthma Immunol 2019;123(2):173–8.e171.

46. Kim Y, Blomberg M, Rifas-Shiman SL, et al. Racial/Ethnic Differences in Incidence and Persistence of Childhood Atopic Dermatitis. J Invest Dermatol 2019;139(4):827–34.

47. Margolis DJ, Gupta J, Apter AJ, et al. Filaggrin-2 variation is associated with more persistent atopic dermatitis in African American subjects. J Allergy Clin Immunol 2014;133(3):784–9.

48. Hong MR, Lei D, Yousaf M, et al. A real-world study of the longitudinal course of adult atopic dermatitis severity in clinical practice. Ann Allergy Asthma Immunol : official publication of the American College of Allergy, Asthma, & Immunology 2020;125(6): 686–92.e683.

49. Zuberbier T, Orlow SJ, Paller AS, et al. Patient perspectives on the management of atopic dermatitis. J Allergy Clin Immunol 2006;118(1):226–32.

50. Chovatiya R, Silverberg JI. Evaluating the Longitudinal Course of Atopic Dermatitis: Implications for Clinical Practice. Am J Clin Dermatol 2022;23(4):459–68.

Global Burden of Atopic Dermatitis
Examining Disease Prevalence Across Pediatric and Adult Populations World-Wide

Kevin Puerta Durango, BS, Zelma C. Chiesa Fuxench, MD, MSCE*

KEYWORDS

• Atopic dermatitis • Eczema • Prevalence • Global

KEY POINTS

• The prevalence of atopic dermatitis (AD) varies widely across the globe.
• AD is thought to be primarily a disease of children, and while studies are more limited, current data suggest that it is also a highly prevalent disease across populations worldwide.
• AD is overall a highly common disease that does not appear to discriminate across populations.

INTRODUCTION

Atopic dermatitis (AD) is a common inflammatory disease associated with marked disease burden and increased health care costs.[1–5] AD is thought to be initially present in childhood with an estimated 60% of children displaying symptoms before 12 months of age, and close to 80% having disease onset before age 6.[6,7] AD is often seen as a disease of children with most patients outgrowing their disease by late childhood.[8] However, increasing evidence supports that AD is highly prevalent in adults and that it is a life-long disease characterized by varying episodes of disease severity throughout a patient's lifetime.[9–11] AD is observed across all ethnicities and can have a profound negative effect on patients and caregivers due to its multidimensional disease burden (**Fig. 1**).[12,13] The purpose of this narrative review is to summarize the most recent data on the global prevalence of AD so that clinicians, patients, and other key stakeholders have a better understanding of the impact of AD across populations.

EPIDEMIOLOGY

A systematic review examining the global prevalence of AD observed an estimated prevalence of approximately 2.6% (95% confidence interval [CI] 1.9, 3.5) or close to 204.05 million people affected. When stratified by age, the prevalence of AD was closer to 2.0% and 4.0% among adults and children, respectively. While the epidemiology of AD varied across geographic regions, 42% of countries lacked reporting of the epidemiologic data underscoring a need for future work in other less-studied countries.[14] (**Fig. 2**).

AFRICA

The prevalence of AD in pediatric cohorts varies greatly across Africa ranging from 0.51% in Tongo to 49.8% in Nigeria.[15–20] In southwestern Nigeria, the prevalence varies from 23% to 27% in school-aged children. Whereas in Senegal, a study of children aged less than 15 years observed an estimated prevalence of 12.2%, and in Ethiopia,

Department of Dermatology, Perelman School of Medicine, University of Pennsylvania, 3400 Civic Center Boulevard, 7th Floor South Tower, Philadelphia, PA 19104, USA
* Corresponding author.
E-mail address: zchi@pennmedicine.upenn.edu

Dermatol Clin 42 (2024) 519–525
https://doi.org/10.1016/j.det.2024.05.004

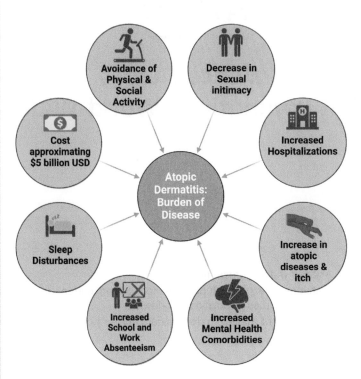

the estimated prevalence of AD among children aged 3 months to 14 years was 9.6% (7.2, 12.5%).[21–23] In a separate, retrospective study in Ghana, AD was the most common diagnosis in infants (0–2 years-old), children (3–12 year-old), and adolescents (13–18 year old) with a prevalence of 31.7%, 30.0%, and 14.9%, respectively.[24] In Botswana, AD was the most common diagnosis in infants (70.7%), preschoolers (61.0%), first schoolers (33.4%), and preadolescents (17.5%) and the third most common among adolescents (10.8%).[25] While studies on the prevalence of AD among adults in Africa are limited, the prevalence among adults in central sub-Saharan Africa has been reported as 2.6% with higher prevalence in females (4.3%) compared to males (3.8%).[14] While in Namibia, the prevalence of AD among adults varied from 16.9% to 24.6%.[26]

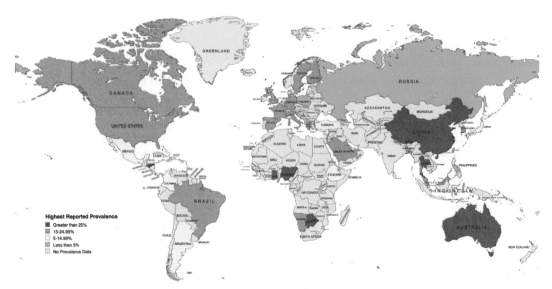

Fig. 2. Worldwide prevalence estimates of Atopic Dermatitis (AD).

MIDDLE EAST, EURASIA, AND EAST ASIA

Studies on the prevalence of AD in Turkey, report AD prevalence ranging from 4.3% to 12.8%.[27,28] A study of school-aged children from ages 7 to 19 years in Saudi Arabia reported AD physician-diagnosed prevalence of 12.5%.[29] While in Israel, the prevalence of AD ranges from 0.9% in children aged less than 6 months to 11.0% among 6 months to 11 years, and 5.8% among those 12 to less than 18 years.[30] Results from the EPI-CARE study, a worldwide, cross-sectional study that examined the 12-month prevalence of AD based on the International Study of Asthma and Allergies in Childhood (ISAAC) criteria and a respondent-reported physician-confirmed diagnosis of AD found an estimated prevalence of 2.7% among children aged less than 18 years in Israel, one of the lowest among all countries surveyed.[31] In Bangladesh, a study that used ISAAC or the United Kingdom Working Party (UKWP) criteria observed an annual prevalence of AD ranging from 2% to 4% to 18% to 20% depending on the criteria used and the pediatric age group under study and a separate study that also relied on ISAAC criteria observed an estimated overall annual prevalence of 11.9% (10.6, 13.3%) among children aged less than 5 years.[32,33] The reported prevalence of AD in Singapore is one of the highest. Findings from a cross-sectional study across households observed an estimated point prevalence of 20.6% in children aged less than 18 years based on UKWP criteria.[34] In a cross-sectional survey of Malaysian children aged 1 to 6 years, observed that the prevalence of AD varied between 12.8% and 16.7%.[35] Similar results were observed in a study from Japan that examined the prevalence of skin diseases over a 10-year period, with AD being the most common skin condition among first graders (12.34%) and the second most common among sixth graders (8.9%).[36] A separate study in a pediatric cohort of Japanese children found an AD lifetime prevalence of 9.9% with lower prevalence in older children compared to younger children and results from the EPI-CARE survey also found a similar prevalence of 10.7%.[31,37] In contrast, AD prevalence is reportedly higher in Korea and China. A study using the data from the 2010 Korean National Health and Nutrition Examination Survey observed a prevalence of 15.0% among children and adolescents, and in China, prevalence estimates vary between 4.76% and 30.48% depending on the population under study and the criteria used for diagnosis.[38–40] In adults across Asia, a cross-sectional survey of ages between 18 and 54 years that met AD UKWP criteria and self-reported a physician's diagnosis of AD, the prevalence varied

from 11.9% to 12.3% in Singapore and Malaysia, to 30.4% in China, and was highest for Thailand at 33.7%.[41] Whereas, a study in China conducted across multiple tertiary care hospitals observed a prevalence of 3.7% to 8.7% among adults depending on geographic location.[42] A cross-sectional study of adults in Saudi Arabia observed an estimated prevalence of physician-diagnosed AD of 13.1% and a separate study that used International Classification of Disease codes for AD observed a similar reported prevalence of 11.8% among adult Saudis.[29,43] Based on UKWP and physician-confirmed diagnosis of AD, the prevalence of AD in Israel has been reported as one of the lowest at 3.4% and a similarly low prevalence has been reported for adults in Russia (4.5%).[41]

EUROPE

Like other regions of the World, prevalence estimates for AD vary across Europe, and while most studies focus on prevalence estimates overall or in children, studies on adolescents and adults are limited.[44] In Spain, the prevalence of AD in adolescents has been reported to be 19.8%.[31] A separate study from Catalonia reported a prevalence of 16.9% among adolescents aged 12 to 17 years while a study of adolescents 14 to 16 years from Valencia observed a lifetime prevalence of 34.9%.[45,46] In northern Greece, the prevalence of pediatric AD was closer to 20.9% and similarly, in France and the United Kingdom (UK), the prevalence of pediatric AD has been reported to be 16.5% in children and adolescents aged 6-months to 18 years, and 18.3% among those 0 to 17 years.[31,47] Similarly, a separate study in the UK also observed a prevalence of 15.3%.[31] In contrast, a study that examined trends of AD prevalence in Italian children aged 0 to 12 years, found that from 2006 to 2012 the prevalence of AD increased from 2.66% to 8.45%.[48] Nevertheless, this was lower than those of a separate study, which observed a prevalence of 17.6%, a difference that could be attributed to variation in the criteria used for AD diagnosis.[31] A study from Poland also observed a lower prevalence of AD across pediatric cohorts (6–7 years: 5.34% and 13–14 years: 4.3%).[49] Whereas AD prevalence in children from Germany has been reported to vary between 7.3% (14–18 years) and 17.13% (0–2 years) with an overall prevalence of 10.35% in children aged less than 18 years.[50] Among adults, a study from the UK observed that the prevalence of AD among various cohorts varied between 7.7% (18–74 years) and 11.6% (75–99 years).[47] A Finnish population-based study observed a lifetime prevalence of 21.9% and a 12-month prevalence of 10.1% in adults aged 30 to 99 years, with prevalence decreasing with age.[51] In a Swedish birth cohort, the prevalence of AD at 24 years of age was 17.8% and the point prevalence of ongoing AD was 8.0% and in Greece, a nationwide cross-sectional study observed a 12-month and lifetime prevalence of AD ranging from 1.7% to 6.4% and 3.7% to 11.4%, respectively.[52]

CENTRAL AND SOUTH AMERICA

Prevalence data for Latin America are more limited compared to other regions. In a cross-sectional study of children aged 1 to 6 years from Bogota, Colombia, the prevalence of AD was 6.5%.[53] A retrospective study using a national claims database from said country observed increasing prevalence rates from 2015 to 2019 (4.23% to 6.77%, respectively), and a separate survey of elementary school-aged children in 2 rural municipalities of Colombia also reported a similar prevalence (6.13%).[54,55] In a population-based survey across 88 municipalities in Brazil that included 6610 households, the prevalence of AD among children less than 12 years ranged from 3.97% to 6.90%, similar to the prevalence reported in ISAAC from a cohort of 23422 Brazilian school-aged children (prevalence of eczema among 6–7 year-old: 8.2%, and 13–14 year-old: 5.0%).[56,57] In contrast, in a separate Brazilian cohort, the 12-months prevalence of AD was closer to 20.1% and ranged from 17.2% to 23.2% in sub-cohorts of children 6 months to less than 6 years and adolescents 12 to less than 18 year-old based on ISAAC criteria.[31] In this same study, the overall 12-month prevalence of AD in children from Colombia, Argentina, and Mexico was 10.8%, 9.7%, and 12.9%, respectively, and a separate study using a modified version of the ISAAC criteria the prevalence of AD during the first year of life was 10.7% and 28.2% in a cohort of infants from El Salvador and Honduras.[58] In a population-based study from Brazil, the prevalence of AD in adults ranged from 0.96% to 1.61% (25–45 years), 0.73%–1.42% (46–60 years), and 0.37%–0.85% (>60 years) while a separate study that relied on UKWP criteria and self-report of physician confirmed diagnosis of AD observed a higher prevalence (9.2%).[41] This same study also observed that the prevalence of AD in adults from Colombia, Argentina, and Mexico was 8.9%, 4.8%, and 9.8%, respectively.[41]

NORTH AMERICA: CANADA AND THE UNITED STATES OF AMERICA

A study using the data from a primary care database from Ontario, Canada observed an AD period prevalence of 3.1% between 2005 and 2015. When separating analysis by age, the AD period prevalence for pediatric patients was 9.9%.[59] In contrast, results of EPI-CARE showed a higher 12-months prevalence of AD (25.4%); however, when the analysis was restricted to children that meet ISAAC criteria and self-report of a physician-confirmed diagnosis of AD the prevalence was closer to 15.1%.[31] Studies that examined the prevalence of AD in adult populations from Canada have also observed lower prevalence compared to pediatric cohorts. For example, a web-based survey in which adults were considered to have AD if they met modified UKWP or ISAAC criteria and self-report of a physician's diagnosis of AD observed a point prevalence of 3.5%. In addition, among adults currently being treated for AD, the prevalence was lower at 2.6%, which is closer to the prevalence reported in a separate study that relied on electronic medical records (1.8%).[9,59]

In the United States (US), a prospective cohort study of mothers and babies with AD observed that the prevalence of AD was 15.0% (11.0%-18.9%), 15.1% (11.5%-18.7%), and 14.5% (10.4%%-18.5%) in children aged 5, 9, and 15 years, respectively.[60] Results from the 2021 National Health Interview Survey (NHIS), a nationally representative survey of the US population reported an overall prevalence of 10.8%.[61] When stratified by age, the prevalence of eczema was 12.1% in children aged 6 to 11 years, followed by 10.4% among children 0 to 5 years of age, and 9.8% in children aged 12 to 17 years.[61] These results are similar to those of the more recent EPI-CARE survey, which observed a prevalence closer to 9.8%.[31] Similar to other countries, the prevalence of AD among US adults is lower compared to pediatric cohorts.[11,62] Two separate population-based studies observed a prevalence closer to 7%. A study that examined the 1-year prevalence of AD among adults using the NHIS reported a prevalence of 7.2%.[62] Whereas a separate study using the data from the Growth from Knowledge (GfK) Knowledge Panel, which relied on modified UKWP criteria for the diagnosis of AD, reported an overall prevalence of 7.3%.[11]

OCEANIA

Few studies have examined the prevalence of AD in populations across countries from the geographic region of Oceania. The data from a population-based database that included 2.1 million patients from 494 primary care practices across Australia observed an overall lifetime and current prevalence of 16.4% and 6.3%, respectively.[63] The prevalence of AD decreased with age in children aged 0 to 4 years having the highest prevalence (lifetime prevalence: 18.8% [17.9, 19.7] and current prevalence: 13.8% [13.1, 14.5]).[63] A separate study that included the data from 4 different cohorts in Australia and Tasmania but used varying definitions to capture eczema or AD diagnosis, observed that in children less than 6 years, the prevalence of ever having eczema varied between 28.8% and 35.6% and the prevalence of current eczema ranged between 16.7% and 26.6%.[64] In this same study, the eczema prevalence ranged between 13.8% and 48.4% across adults while the 1-year prevalence was 15.1% at age 18 but decreased to 8.8% by age 53.[64] A separate study observed that the lifetime prevalence and current prevalence of AD was lowest among ages 30 to 34 years (lifetime prevalence: 11.6% [10.9, 12.2] and current prevalence: 5.0 [4.8, 5.3]) and highest among ages 85 to 89 years (lifetime prevalence: 24.8 [23.5, 26.2]) and 80 to 84 years (current prevalence: 8.0 [7.4, 8.6]).[63]

In summary, AD is a highly prevalent disease worldwide in both pediatric and adult populations. Studies that examine differences in prevalence across populations may be difficult to compare due to differences in study designs including how AD is diagnosed. Despite these limitations, understanding the full burden of AD is critical if the authors are to improve the lives of patients and caregivers living with AD and gain a broader understanding of impact of AD across the globe.

CLINICS CARE POINTS

- AD is a highly prevalent disease in children and adults worldwide.
- While AD is not thought to discriminate across populations, worldwide prevalence estimates vary greatly.
- Understanding the full burden of AD including the societal impacts of this disease is critical to improving the care and quality of life of patients with AD.

DISCLOSURE

Z.C. Chiesa Fuxench has received research grants from Lilly, United States, LEO Pharma, Denmark, Brexogen, Regeneron, United States, Sanofi, United States, Tioga, and Vanda, United States for work related to Atopic Dermatitis and from Menlo Therapeutics and Galderma for work related to prurigo nodularis. She has also served as consultant for the Asthma and Allergy Foundation of America, National Eczema Association, AbbVie, Incyte Corporation, and Pfizer; and received honoraria for CME work in Atopic Dermatitis sponsored by education grants from Regeneron/Sanofi and Pfizer, United States and from Beirsdorf for work related to skin cancer and sun protection. K. Puerta Durango has no interests to disclose.

REFERENCES

1. Laughter MR, Maymone MBC, Mashayekhi S, et al. The global burden of atopic dermatitis: lessons from the Global Burden of Disease Study 1990-2017. Br J Dermatol 2021;184(2):304–9.
2. Peng C, Yu N, Ding Y, et al. Epidemiological variations in global burden of atopic dermatitis: An analysis of trends from 1990 to 2019. Allergy 2022;77(9):2843–5.
3. Shin YH, Hwang J, Kwon R, et al. Global, regional, and national burden of allergic disorders and their risk factors in 204 countries and territories, from 1990 to 2019: A systematic analysis for the Global Burden of Disease Study 2019. Allergy 2023;78(8):2232–54.
4. Eyerich K, Gooderham MJ, Silvestre JF, et al. Real-world clinical, psychosocial and economic burden of atopic dermatitis: Results from a multicountry study. J Eur Acad Dermatol Venereol 2023. https://doi.org/10.1111/jdv.19500.
5. Capozza K, Funk M, Hering M, et al. Patients' and caregivers' experiences with atopic dermatitis-related burden, medical care, and treatments in 8 countries. J Allergy Clin Immunol Pract 2023;11(1):264–73.e1.
6. Eichenfield LF, Stripling S, Fung S, et al. Recent developments and advances in atopic dermatitis: a focus on epidemiology, pathophysiology, and treatment in the pediatric setting. Paediatr Drugs 2022;24(4):293–305.
7. Weidinger S, Beck LA, Bieber T, et al. Atopic dermatitis. Nat Rev Dis Primers 2018;4(1):1.
8. Pyun BY. Natural history and risk factors of atopic dermatitis in children. Allergy Asthma Immunol Res 2015;7(2):101–5.
9. Barbarot S, Auziere S, Gadkari A, et al. Epidemiology of atopic dermatitis in adults: Results from an international survey. Allergy 2018;73(6):1284–93.
10. Abuabara K, Margolis DJ, Langan SM. The long-term course of atopic dermatitis. Dermatol Clin 2017;35(3):291–7.
11. Chiesa Fuxench ZC, Block JK, Boguniewicz M, et al. Atopic dermatitis in america study: a cross-sectional study examining the prevalence and disease burden of atopic dermatitis in the US Adult Population. J Invest Dermatol 2019;139(3):583–90.
12. Bridgman AC, Block JK, Drucker AM. The multidimensional burden of atopic dermatitis: An update. Ann Allergy Asthma Immunol 2018;120(6):603–6.

13. Worldwide variation in prevalence of symptoms of asthma, allergic rhinoconjunctivitis, and atopic eczema: ISAAC. The International Study of Asthma and Allergies in Childhood (ISAAC) Steering Committee. Lancet 1998;351(9111):1225–32.

14. Tian J, Zhang D, Yang Y, et al. Global epidemiology of atopic dermatitis: a comprehensive systematic analysis and modelling study. Br J Dermatol 2023; 190(1):55–61.

15. Ayanlowo O, Puddicombe O, Gold-Olufadi S. Pattern of skin diseases amongst children attending a dermatology clinic in Lagos, Nigeria. Pan Afr Med J 2018;29:162.

16. Akinboro AO, Mejiuni AD, Akinlade MO, et al. Spectrum of skin diseases presented at LAUTECH Teaching Hospital, Osogbo, southwest Nigeria. Int J Dermatol 2015;54(4):443–50.

17. Wey GD, Adefemi SA, Amao EA. Prevalence and pattern of atopic dermatitis among children aged 6 months to 14 years seen in general out-patient clinic of federal medical centre, bida. West Afr J Med Apr-2020;37(2):124–30.

18. Ewurum O, Ibeneme CA, Nnaji TO, et al. Spectrum of skin disorders among primary school children in Umuahia, South-East Nigeria. Niger J Clin Pract 2022;25(7):1076–82.

19. Oninla OA, Oninla SO, Onayemi O, et al. Pattern of paediatric dermatoses at dermatology clinics in Ile-Ife and Ilesha, Nigeria. Paediatr Int Child Health 2016;36(2):106–12.

20. Clessou JNT, Dovi-Tevi KA, Kombate K, et al. [Distribution of dermatoses encountered in children seen in Dermatological Consultations in Lome (Togo)]. Med Trop Sante Int 2022;2(2). Distribution des dermatoses rencontrees chez les enfants vus en Consultation Dermatologique a Lome (Togo).

21. Kayode OA, Mokoatle CM, Rathebe PC, et al. Factors Associated with Atopic Dermatitis among Children Aged 6 to 14 Years in Alimosho Local Government, Lagos, Nigeria. Children 2023;10(5).

22. Herrant M, Loucoubar C, Boufkhed S, et al. Risk factors associated with asthma, atopic dermatitis and rhinoconjunctivitis in a rural Senegalese cohort. Allergy Asthma Clin Immunol 2015;11(1):24.

23. Kelbore AG, Alemu W, Shumye A, et al. Magnitude and associated factors of Atopic dermatitis among children in Ayder referral hospital, Mekelle, Ethiopia. BMC Dermatol 2015;15:15.

24. Rosenbaum BE, Klein R, Hagan PG, et al. Dermatology in Ghana: a retrospective review of skin disease at the Korle Bu Teaching Hospital Dermatology Clinic. Pan Afr Med J 2017;26:125.

25. Sethomo W, Williams VL, Tladi P, et al. Skin conditions among pediatric dermatology outpatients in Botswana. Pediatr Dermatol 2022;39(6):883–8.

26. Munyaradzi Mukesi INP, Moyo Sylvester R, Mtambo Owen PL. Prevalence of skin allergies in adolescents in namibia. International Journal of Allergy Medications 2017;3(1).

27. Aksoy AG, Boran P, Karakoc-Aydiner E, et al. Prevalence of allergic disorders and risk factors associated with food allergy in Turkish preschoolers. Allergol Immunopathol 2021;49(1):11–6.

28. Dogruel D, Bingol G, Altintas DU, et al. Prevalence of and risk factors for atopic dermatitis: A birth cohort study of infants in southeast Turkey. Allergol Immunopathol May-2016;44(3):214–20.

29. Alqahtani JM. Asthma and other allergic diseases among Saudi schoolchildren in Najran: the need for a comprehensive intervention program. Ann Saudi Med Nov-2016;36(6):379–85.

30. Weil C, Sugerman PB, Chodick G, et al. Epidemiology and economic burden of atopic dermatitis: real-world retrospective data from a large nationwide israeli healthcare provider database. Adv Ther 2022;39(6):2502–14.

31. Silverberg JI, Barbarot S, Gadkari A, et al. Atopic dermatitis in the pediatric population: A cross-sectional, international epidemiologic study. Ann Allergy Asthma Immunol 2021;126(4):417–28.e2.

32. Pedersen CJ, Uddin MJ, Saha SK, et al. Prevalence of atopic dermatitis, asthma and rhinitis from infancy through adulthood in rural Bangladesh: a population-based, cross-sectional survey. BMJ Open 2020; 10(11):e042380.

33. Pedersen CJ, Uddin MJ, Saha SK, et al. Prevalence and psychosocial impact of atopic dermatitis in Bangladeshi children and families. PLoS One 2021; 16(4):e0249824.

34. Cheok S, Yee F, Song Ma JY, et al. Prevalence and descriptive epidemiology of atopic dermatitis and its impact on quality of life in Singapore. Br J Dermatol 2018;178(1):276–7.

35. Goh YY, Keshavarzi F, Chew YL. Prevalence of Atopic Dermatitis and Pattern of Drug Therapy in Malaysian Children. Dermatitis May/2018;29(3):151–61.

36. Tanaka A, Niimi N, Takahashi M, et al. Prevalence of skin diseases and prognosis of atopic dermatitis in primary school children in populated areas of Japan from 2010 to 2019: The Asa Study in Hiroshima, Japan. J Dermatol 2022;49(12):1284–90.

37. Okada Y, Kumagai H, Morikawa Y, et al. Epidemiology of pediatric allergic diseases in the Ogasawara Islands. Allergol Int 2016;65(1):37–43.

38. Lee KS, Oh IH, Choi SH, et al. Analysis of epidemiology and risk factors of atopic dermatitis in korean children and adolescents from the 2010 Korean National Health and Nutrition Examination Survey. BioMed Res Int 2017;2017:5142754.

39. Guo Y, Li P, Tang J, et al. Prevalence of atopic dermatitis in chinese children aged 1-7 ys. Sci Rep 2016;6:29751.

40. Liu Y, Sun S, Zhang D, et al. Effects of residential environment and lifestyle on atopic eczema among

preschool children in Shenzhen, China. Front Public Health 2022;10:844832.

41. Maspero J, De Paula Motta Rubini N, Zhang J, et al. Epidemiology of adult patients with atopic dermatitis in AWARE 1: A second international survey. World Allergy Organ J 2023;16(3):100724.

42. Wang X, Shi XD, Li LF, et al. Prevalence and clinical features of adult atopic dermatitis in tertiary hospitals of China. Medicine (Baltim) 2017;96(11):e6317.

43. Alshamrani HM, Alsolami MA, Alshehri AM, et al. Pattern of skin diseases in a university hospital in Jeddah, Saudi Arabia: age and sex distribution. Ann Saudi Med Jan-2019;39(1):22–8.

44. Bylund S, Kobyletzki LB, Svalstedt M, et al. Prevalence and incidence of atopic dermatitis: a systematic review. Acta Derm Venereol 2020;100(12):adv00160.

45. Arnedo-Pena A, Puig-Barbera J, Artero-Civera A, et al. Atopic dermatitis incidence and risk factors in young adults in Castellon (Spain): A prospective cohort study. Allergol Immunopathol Nov-2020; 48(6):694–700.

46. Mora T, Sanchez-Collado I, Mullol J, et al. Prevalence of atopic dermatitis in the adolescent population of Catalonia (Spain). Allergol Immunopathol 2023;51(4):101–9.

47. Chan LN, Magyari A, Ye M, et al. The epidemiology of atopic dermatitis in older adults: A population-based study in the United Kingdom. PLoS One 2021;16(10):e0258219.

48. Cantarutti A, Dona D, Visentin F, et al. Epidemiology of frequently occurring skin diseases in italian children from 2006 to 2012: a retrospective, population-based study. Pediatr Dermatol Sep-2015;32(5): 668–78.

49. Sybilski AJ, Raciborski F, Lipiec A, et al. Atopic dermatitis is a serious health problem in Poland. Epidemiology studies based on the ECAP study. Postepy Dermatol Alergol 2015;32(1):1–10.

50. Augustin M, Radtke MA, Glaeske G, et al. Epidemiology and Comorbidity in Children with Psoriasis and Atopic Eczema. Dermatology 2015;231(1):35–40.

51. Kiiski V, Salava A, Susitaival P, et al. Atopic dermatitis in adults: a population-based study in Finland. Int J Dermatol 2022;61(3):324–30.

52. Stefanou G, Gregoriou S, Kontodimas S, et al. Prevalence of adult self-reported atopic dermatitis in Greece: results from a nationwide survey. Eur J Dermatol 2022;32(5):597–606. Prevalence of adult self-reported atopic dermatitis in Greece: results from a nationwide survey.

53. Garcia E, Halpert E, Borrero E, et al. Prevalence of skin diseases in children 1 to 6 years old in the city of Bogota, Colombia. World Allergy Organ J 2020;13(12):100484.

54. Londono AM, Castro-Ayarza JR, Kronfly A, et al. Epidemiology and healthcare resource utilization in atopic dermatitis in Colombia: A retrospective analysis of data from the National Health Registry from 2015 to 2020. Biomedica 2023;43(1):107–20. Epidemiologia y uso de recursos de salud en dermatitis atopica en Colombia: analisis retrospectivo de datos del Registro Nacional de Salud de 2015 a 2020.

55. Moreno-Lopez S, Perez-Herrera LC, Penaranda D, et al. Prevalence and associated factors of allergic diseases in school children and adolescents aged 6-7 and 13-14 years from two rural areas in Colombia. Allergol Immunopathol 2021;49(3):153–61.

56. Miot HA, Aoki V, Orfali RL, et al. The (one-year) prevalence of atopic dermatitis in Brazil: A population-based telephone survey. J Eur Acad Dermatol Venereol 2023. https://doi.org/10.1111/jdv. 19071.

57. Solé D, Camelo-Nunes IC, Wandalsen GF, et al. Prevalence of atopic eczema and related symptoms in Brazilian schoolchildren: results from the International Study of Asthma and Allergies in Childhood (ISAAC) phase 3. J Investig Allergol Clin Immunol 2006;16(6):367–76.

58. Draaisma E, Garcia-Marcos L, Mallol J, et al. A multinational study to compare prevalence of atopic dermatitis in the first year of life. Pediatr Allergy Immunol 2015;26(4):359–66.

59. Drucker AM, Bai L, Eder L, et al. Sociodemographic characteristics and emergency department visits and inpatient hospitalizations for atopic dermatitis in Ontario: a cross-sectional study. CMAJ Open 2022;10(2):E491–9.

60. McKenzie C, Silverberg JI. The prevalence and persistence of atopic dermatitis in urban United States children. Ann Allergy Asthma Immunol 2019;123(2):173–8.e1.

61. Zablotsky B, Black LI, Akinbami LJ. Diagnosed allergic conditions in children aged 0-17 Years: United States, 2021. NCHS Data Brief 2023;459:1–8.

62. Hua T, Silverberg JI. Atopic dermatitis in US adults: Epidemiology, association with marital status, and atopy. Ann Allergy Asthma Immunol 2018;121(5): 622–4.

63. Chidwick K, Busingye D, Pollack A, et al. Prevalence, incidence and management of atopic dermatitis in Australian general practice using routinely collected data from MedicineInsight. Australas J Dermatol 2020;61(3):e319–27.

64. Zeleke BM, Lowe AJ, Dharmage SC, et al. Epidemiology of eczema in South-Eastern Australia. Australas J Dermatol 2023;64(1):e41–50.

The Role of Food Allergy in Atopic Dermatitis

Brit Trogen, MD, MS[a], Megha Verma, DO[b], Scott H. Sicherer, MD[a], Amanda Cox, MD[a],*

KEYWORDS

• Atopic dermatitis • Food allergy • Sensitization • Dietary interventions • Immunologic mechanisms

KEY POINTS

• Many individuals are affected by both atopic dermatitis (AD) and IgE-mediated food allergy simultaneously.
• There is keen interest in whether there is a causal relationship between AD and food allergy.
• In general, AD is a risk factor for the development of food allergy, while food allergy is rarely a cause of AD.
• Sensitization to foods is common in patients with AD, and can lead to the overdiagnosis and/or misdiagnosis of food allergy.
• Dietary elimination of allergenic foods can have unintended harmful effects, including the development of immediate-type allergy to previously tolerated foods.

THE RELATIONSHIP BETWEEN ATOPIC DERMATITIS AND FOOD ALLERGY

Atopic dermatitis (AD) is a chronic inflammatory skin condition characterized by intense pruritus and recurrent eczematous skin lesions. It is the most common inflammatory skin disorder in childhood, affecting up to 20% of children and 3% to 10% of adults.[1,2] Any clinician who has encountered this disease has likely witnessed the immense negative consequences it can have for the quality of life, sleep quality, development, and functioning of affected patients and their families.[1] Despite the connotation "atopic," AD is not necessarily an allergic disease and occurs often in individuals who are not sensitized to food or environmental allergens.[3] However, rates of allergic disorders in patients with AD are substantial, with up to 80% of affected children going on to develop other atopic conditions, which include allergic rhinitis and asthma later in life, in a progression often termed the "atopic march."[4,5] Furthermore, the presence of early childhood AD is recognized as a strong risk factor for the development of food allergy.[6]

The relationship between AD and food allergy is complex, and whether one condition causes the other has been a topic of controversy.[7] An understanding of the interplay between skin inflammation and AD control, as well as cutaneous and oral exposure to foods, is crucial for evaluating and managing young patients with AD who may have food allergy. The onset of AD and the development of food allergy may coincide early in life. Atopic dermatitis often emerges in infancy just as a wide range of foods are being introduced in the diet. Because AD typically waxes and wanes, with exacerbations and periods of improvement, it may appear that the development of and severity of eczema is related to foods ingested by an infant or nursing mother. Often, parents of affected infants eliminate many foods in attempts to achieve control of AD, almost always without observed clinical improvement. Some foods such as acidic fruits and certain spices can act as irritants and cause rash in those with sensitive skin and flares

a Division of Pediatric Allergy, Icahn School of Medicine at Mount Sinai, One Gustave Levy Place, New York, NY 10029, USA; b Department of Internal Medicine, Mount Sinai Morningside/West, 1111 Amsterdam Avenue, New York, NY 10025, USA
* Corresponding author.
E-mail address: amanda.cox@mssm.edu

Dermatol Clin 42 (2024) 527–535
https://doi.org/10.1016/j.det.2024.04.004
0733-8635/24/

in those with AD, and may be mistaken by patients and families as food allergens. Immunoglobulin (Ig) E-mediated food allergy is present in a subset of patients with AD, and allergic reactions to foods can trigger AD exacerbations; however, food allergy is rarely the underlying or sole cause of AD, and there are risks posed by to elimination diets in young patients with AD.[7,8]

In examining the relationship between AD and food allergy, it is important to clarify the distinction between "sensitization" and clinically relevant "allergy" to foods.[9] Sensitization is the production of IgE to a specific food by the cells of the immune system; a person would be "sensitized" to milk if milk-specific IgE is detected in their serum or if percutaneous skin testing to milk produces a 3 mm or larger wheal. However, allergy is present if there is a clinical reaction upon exposure to the food. A person could be sensitized to a food, yet eat it regularly without issue—and in fact, many do. In the setting of sensitization to tolerated foods, food elimination, or avoidance may increase individual risk of developing food allergy that may not otherwise have manifested, a point that will be discussed in greater depth later in this section.

There are increased rates of food sensitization in individuals with atopic dermatitis.[8] The general elevation in total serum IgE often seen in this population, especially when eczema is in a highly inflamed state, can result in elevated allergen-specific IgE that typically has no clinical significance.[10,11] A recent systematic review and meta-analysis found that pooled prevalence of food sensitization, food allergy, and challenge-proven food allergy among 225,568 individuals with AD was 48.4%, 32.7%, and 40.7%, respectively.[12] This was significantly higher than the prevalence of these conditions among those without AD, who reported pooled prevalence of 17.9%, 9.4%, and 15.5%, respectively. Children with AD had higher pooled food sensitization and food allergy than adults (49.8% and 31.4%, compared with 28.6% and 24.1%), again suggesting a stronger link in the early years of life. The highest pooled prevalence of food sensitization and food allergy in individuals with AD was found at 0 to 2 years of age, to be 54.4% and 39.2%, respectively.

Based on these abundance of data, it seems clear that atopic dermatitis, particularly when it emerges early in life, is a significant risk factor for food allergy.[7]

The gold standard for diagnosing food allergy is the double-blind, placebo-controlled oral food challenge (DBPCFC), and has been examined in studies to determine the true prevalence of IgE-mediated food allergy among infants and children with AD. IgE-mediated food allergy in this population ranges from 33% to 63% across several studies (though importantly, these studies excluded those who reported anaphylactic reactions or who had positive food-specific IgE elevated in a range typically diagnostic of allergy)[13–15]; These rates exceed the prevalence of food allergy in the general pediatric population, which was recently estimated at 7.6% based on a survey of 38,408 United States (US) households, and provides further evidence for AD as a risk factor for food allergy.[12,16] This finding was reiterated in HealthNuts, a large Australian study in which 20% of children with AD demonstrated allergy by oral food challenge (OFC) to peanut, egg white, or sesame seed, in comparison to 4% of children without eczema.[17]

Many of these studies highlight that age of onset and severity of eczema contributes to food allergy development, with earlier onset and more severe eczema augering greater allergy risk. Children with onset of AD before 3 months of age, for instance, have a significantly higher association with positive egg, milk, and peanut-specific-IgE.[18] In HealthNuts, one-year-old infants with eczema were 11 times more likely to have peanut allergy, and 6 times more likely to have egg allergy than children without eczema. Severity of disease is also a strong predictor of the development of both sensitization and allergy to foods, with more severe AD resulting in substantially greater rates of sensitization and allergy.[18,19]

IMMUNOLOGIC MECHANISMS LINKING ATOPIC DERMATITIS AND FOOD ALLERGY

The complex pathophysiology of AD involves the interplay of several factors including genetic predisposition, dysfunction of the epidermal barrier, and inflammation driven by T-cells.[20] While the immunologic mechanisms that link atopic and dermatitis are not fully understood, both involve a shared immunologic pathway that is associated with elevated serum IgE and a T-helper type 2 (Th2) response.[20–22] However, while AD has classically been considered a largely Th2-driven response, other T cells including Th1, Th17, and Th22 are now also known to contribute to AD pathogenesis, and different endotypes of AD are being identified with varying involvement of these cell classes.[23] Inflammation of the skin in AD is associated with the release of interleukin-4 (IL-4), interleukin-13(IL-13), and thymic stromal lymphopoietin (TSLP), all of which result in Th2 inflammation, Ig class switching, and higher IgE levels.[20,24] Among other atopic diseases, AD is associated more elevated average total serum IgE levels, typically more than normal and in 100s to 1000s kU/L range. One hypothesis is that elevated total serum IgE in AD increases the likelihood of the production of food-specific IgE (sensitization) and the development of food allergy. Serum IgE levels have also been shown to be influenced by genetic modifications, in particular IL-13 variants.[25] IL-13 variants can result in higher total serum IgE levels, as well as sensitization to specific food allergens, most commonly hen's egg, in young children with AD.[26]

The epidermal barrier in AD demonstrates many functional defects including poor water retention, decreased ceramide lipid content, and reduced protective proteins such as filaggrin (FLG).[24] The dysfunction of the skin barrier in AD may in turn play a significant role in the development of food allergy and has been supported by several observations in studies. Individuals with a loss-of-function FLG mutation have a 3 to 5 times higher risk of AD, and are predisposed to develop aeroallergen sensitization, food allergy and asthma.[27–29]

The disrupted epidermal barrier may be particularly important in the development of food allergy in infants and young children with atopic dermatitis. While historically it was believed that sensitization to food allergens occurred primarily via allergen exposure in the gut, there is increasing evidence that sensitization can occur, and is significantly more likely to occur following primary allergen exposure on the skin. Moreover, this effect may be amplified in the setting of inflammation and impaired skin barrier that are characteristic of AD. One study supporting this found an increased rate of peanut sensitization with environmental exposure to peanut measured in living room dust in children with a history of AD.[30] Additional evidence of a skin route for peanut sensitization was demonstrated by a study in which the rate of peanut allergy was not affected by infant oral exposure to peanut but was increased in infants for whom topical creams containing peanut oil had been applied to inflamed skin before 6 months of age.[19] Another example of skin barrier dysfunction contributing to allergic sensitization is exemplified by the findings that mutations in the serine peptidase inhibitor Kazal type 5 genes are associated with asthma, AD, and with challenge-proven IgE-mediated food allergy, as noted in the Netherton Syndrome.[31] Further indication that skin barrier integrity may be a factor in food allergy development is illustrated by a retrospective study of infants under 1 year of age, for whom aggressive use of topical corticosteroid to shorten the course of eczema resulted in decreased food allergy development.[32]

DERMATOLOGIC CLINICAL MANIFESTATIONS OF FOOD ALLERGY

In an IgE-mediated allergic reaction to food, cutaneous symptoms may include acute (within minutes to hours) onset of urticaria, pruritus, angioedema, erythroderma, and flushing, and may or may not be associated with respiratory, gastrointestinal, circulatory or neurologic symptoms of a systemic allergic reaction.[33] Neither AD-onset and flares are typical of an acute allergic reaction nor is AD a hallmark of anaphylaxis. AD can develop following acute pruritus and scratching within 2 hours of an immediate allergic food reaction, or may not manifest until 6 to 48 hours later.[34,35] In 1985, Sampson *and colleagues* established that AD is linked to IgE-mediated food allergy in a study of 101 positive DBPCFCs in 113 children with severe AD.[36] While older studies of DBPCFCs have demonstrated that AD in children can be exacerbated by a food, it is not clear how often AD was observed as the only symptom.[7] Nonetheless, the most commonly implicated foods linked to worsening eczema, have been cow's milk, egg, and peanut.[7,37] One European study implicated birch pollen-related foods such as apple, carrot, hazelnut, and celery as AD triggers.[38] A more recent Dutch study looking at 1186 DBPCFCs in 682 children, did not identify AD or eczema flares to be common manifestations of food reactions.[35] These investigators found that children with AD were more frequently sensitized to food without clinical reactions compared with those without AD. Furthermore, they concluded that a child is unlikely to have an allergy to a food if the only symptom observed or reported following food ingestion or food challenge is AD. For adults, a causal link between AD and food allergy has not been well-studied or described.

In summary, the relationship between food allergy and AD is likely more impacted by AD being a risk factor for developing food allergy and not that food allergy is a trigger for developing or exacerbating AD. An understanding of this relationship has significant implications for the clinical management of AD, in particular with regard to food allergy testing, skin care, and dietary management, and has informed recently published practice parameters.[39]

To illustrate the diagnostic challenges of these conditions, the authors have prepared the following hypothetical cases, based on commonly encountered clinical scenarios.

- Case 1: A 9-month-old has a history of AD that initially developed around 2 to 3 months of age involving the cheeks, abdomen, and neck. The infant was initially introduced to scrambled eggs around 6 months of age without immediate adverse reactions, and continued to eat eggs every 2 to 3 days for the next month. However, the infant's parents noticed worsening of eczema beginning around 6 months of age, despite treatment with prescription topical steroid. Allergy evaluation conducted at 7 months of age demonstrated egg sensitization, with negative skin prick testing but serum egg white specific IgE of 0.44 kU/L. The family decided to eliminate egg from the diet because of concerns about egg as possible triggers for eczema. Over the 3 months during which egg was avoided, the eczema significantly improved. However, at 9 months of age, within minutes of trying egg in the form of French toast, the patient experienced acute respiratory distress, facial swelling, and hives, requiring prompt treatment by family with intramuscular epinephrine, and transport to an emergency department for continued observation. Subsequent allergy testing at 10 months of age demonstrated egg white serum specific IgE of 12.2 kU/L and ovomucoid IgE of 9.4 kU/L. The family was advised to strictly avoid all forms of egg and to carry an epinephrine auto-injector at all times.

Case 2: A 3-year-old presented in early infancy with AD and their primary care provider tested the child and documented multiple food sensitizations by serum IgE laboratory testing. Based on this testing, any foods with positive tests were not introduced, and the family had been avoiding dairy, soy, wheat, peanuts, and tree nuts. In part due to these restrictions, the child demonstrated poor weight gain, picky eating, and developed vitamin D deficiency. At 3 years, the eczema was moderately well-controlled on a regimen of topical steroids and frequent emollient use. Testing for avoided foods were repeated, and over the course of 2.5 years, the patient passed allergist-supervised OFCs to soy, wheat, dairy, peanut, and almond, prompting introduction of the previously avoided foods, and dramatically improving the options for a diverse diet. There are plans to complete food challenges for the remaining tree nuts. The patient's parents, in collaboration with a pediatric allergist and dietician, continue to implement nutritional supplementation, feeding therapy, and offer a balanced diet to address his low weight.

As these cases demonstrate, it can be difficult to tease out the complex interplay of cause and effect between AD and food allergy, and hard to navigate the diagnostic and management challenges these conditions pose. The potential harms of allergy testing in the absence of prior clinical allergic reactions must also be carefully considered in this patient population.

Food-specific serum IgE levels and skin prick tests to individual foods cannot distinguish between food sensitization and clinical allergy, whereas observing an individual ingesting a food, either through home introduction or supervised OFC, provides the best evidence of tolerance versus allergy. During an OFC, skin manifestations are one of several objective clinical signs of allergy, which should be monitored. In a patient with underlying eczematous dermatitis, however, some skin symptoms can be difficult to interpret. Skin symptoms during a food challenge that consist only of worsening eczema or AD, possibly manifesting as increased erythema or pruritus of existing eczematous patches of skin, in the absence of urticaria, angioedema, or other immediate-type symptoms, can be confounding. If a patient's reaction during an OFC is limited to an eczema flare, is this a sufficient indicator of a positive OFC, and should the patient continue strict avoidance of a food? One early landmark study of children with severe AD found that 84% demonstrated cutaneous symptoms during oral food challenge, making this far from theoretic.[36] Also complicating the interpretation of eczema flares as a sign of food allergy is the phenomenon of skin erythema and pruritus that can result from the acidity of citrus fruits, tomato, and strawberries, as well as from any food having direct skin contact with the perioral region for many infants. Knowledge of the aforementioned confounders and pitfalls, as well as familiarity with the nature of a particular patient's eczema, should be considered during observation and interpretation of an OFC for a patient with underlying or active AD.

PRENATAL DIET, INFANT FORMULA, AND SUPPLEMENTS

There has been keen interest regarding whether the maternal diet during pregnancy and lactation, as well as whether formula choice and vitamin or probiotic supplementation may play a role in preventing or treating atopic dermatitis.[40] A 2008 Association of American Publishers (AAP) report, and 3 follow-up systematic reviews have concluded from published studies that exclusion of foods such as milk, egg, peanut, tree nuts, and fish during pregnancy or while breastfeeding do not prevent AD, including AD, in infants.[41] Furthermore studies of the effects of maternal dietary elimination during breastfeeding on infants who already have AD are limited and have shown conflicting results, thus further research is needed.

Even without considering the maternal diet, breast milk by itself has been investigated for potential protective and beneficial effects with respect to all childhood atopic diseases, including AD. The evidence is not strong, but does suggest that there is an AD prevention benefit to exclusive breastfeeding for 3 to 4 months (but not beyond 4 months) for those with a first-degree family history of AD.[42–44] Numerous studies have also examined whether formula choice may impact the development of atopic disease, and results have been conflicting. Current consensus is that there is insufficient evidence that hydrolyzed or partially-hydrolyzed formulas prevent AD even in those who are considered high-risk for atopy, and this is reflected in the most recent AAP clinical report.[40] Furthermore, soy formula has not been shown to prevent atopy, and amino-acid elemental formulas have not been studied for their preventative effects.[45] Regarding essential fatty acids, which have anti-inflammatory properties; studies have not yet demonstrated convincing benefit for infant AD by maternal supplementation with omega-3, omega-6 fatty acids or evening primrose oil during lactation.[46]

Many studies have focused on supplementation for infants at risk of developing AD, as well as for children with AD, but so far results are not conclusive. A meta-analysis has shown that serum vitamin D is lower in patients with AD, and in particular for those with more severe AD, and vitamin D supplementation has been examined for potential therapeutic benefit in AD.[47] Furthermore, there has been considerable exploration of probiotics, in particular *Lactobacillus* and *Bifidobacteria*, and prebiotics, for their microbiome modulating and anti-inflammatory effects, and possible role in preventing or treating AD. A 2018 Cochrane review of 39 randomized controlled trials did not find that probiotics reduced the severity of eczema,[48] while there is some evidence from studies that prenatal and postnatal probiotics may reduce the risk of infants developing AD.[49] Given the heterogeneity of these studies, however, it is difficult to make conclusions about the preventative or therapeutic effects on AD, and there is no evidence-based recommendation about vitamin D supplementation, probiotics, or prebiotics at this time for breastfeeding parents and infants.

PREVENTION AND MANAGEMENT OF ATOPIC DERMATITIS AND FOOD ALLERGY

Optimization of skin care practices, including avoidance of irritants, aggressive moisturizer application, and the use of topical anti-inflammatory medication, is a cornerstone of the management of AD, and is recommended as the first-line therapy before considering food allergy testing or intervention.[7] However, it is unclear if aggressive treatment of AD may aid in preventing food allergy. Given the evidence for epicutaneous sensitization through a dysfunctional skin barrier, it has been hypothesized that moisturizer used to restore the skin barrier in AD, may reduce allergic sensitization.[2] In one study, early aggressive application of topical corticosteroids to shorten the duration of eczema followed by frequent emollient use in infants with AD was associated with a decrease in later development of food allergies.[32] A subsequent prospective, randomized controlled trial failed to replicate this finding, and in fact demonstrated the opposite finding: In the Enquiring About Tolerance study population, regular application of moisturizers to young infants' skin was associated with increased development of food allergy.[50] The reasons for this are unclear, and could potentially reflect increased likelihood of cutaneous exposure if food proteins are also present during moisturizing, or may indicate inappropriate moisturizer selection. However, studies have not produced conclusive evidence regarding whether moisturizer type, frequency, and age at application can contribute to preventing the development of food allergies.[2]

The recently published 2023 AD guidelines recommend against the use of elimination diets as an intervention for treatment of AD.[39] This stems from the potential risks of food elimination causing the development of IgE-mediated allergy, particularly for infants, as well as the risk of causing malnutrition as a result of dietary restriction. A systematic meta-analysis of dietary elimination for AD included 10 trials (599 patients, mean age of 1.5 years) that examined the harms and benefits of elimination diets for the treatment of AD.[51] The investigators concluded that elimination diets may lead to a slight but unimportant improvement in eczema severity, pruritus, and sleep disorder in those with mild to moderate AD. They also noted indirect evidence of an increased risk of development of peanut allergy when peanut was eliminated from the diets of infants with severe AD until age 5.[52] In a review of 298 pediatric patients with suspected food-triggered AD who underwent elimination diets, 19% went on to develop new immediate-type food reactions and 30% of these reactions were anaphylaxis.[53] In addition to the potential for an elimination diet to increase the likelihood of IgE-mediated food allergy, the 2023 AD guidelines panel proposed that additional harms of an elimination diet could include malnutrition and undue burden for patients and caregivers.[39] They also stated that more research is needed to clarify the interplay between dietary elimination and the immunologic mechanisms that result in eczema flares because of food allergens. Evidence and expert guidance overall suggest that elimination of food from the diet to treat AD should be discouraged.

By contrast, early introduction of allergenic foods such as peanut and egg has been shown to significantly reduce the risk of FA in young infants, and many food allergy prevention guidelines now recommend this approach.[54] The data on AD with respect to food introduction are more mixed. One case-control study found that early solid food introduction before 4 months of age was associated with lower risk of AD reported via parent questionnaire.[55] However, other prospective cohort studies have found no difference, positive or negative, in rates of AD associated with timing of solid food introduction.[56,57] Overall, early food introduction remains a mainstay of FA prevention and should be recommended in accordance with current guidelines.

Finally, biologic medications have emerged as promising therapeutic options for the treatment of many allergic conditions, including asthma, chronic urticaria, nasal polyposis, eosinophilic gastrointestinal disease, atopic dermatitis, and food allergy. Rather than targeting individual allergens, these medications target specific molecular mechanisms that drive allergic reactions, in particular by inhibiting T_H2 T-cell, and some non-T_H2 cell, activation pathways. As a result, biologic agents offer a more targeted approach compared with traditional treatments, as well as the potential to treat multiple coexisting disease states at once.[58] With the recognition that the pathogenesis of both AD and food allergy involve skin barrier defects and type 2 allergic inflammation, some of the same agents are being investigated for both conditions.[59] In particular, biologics targeting IgE, IL-4, and IL-13, and alarmins (TSLP, IL-33, and IL-25), appear to be closest to clinical implementation.[58]

Of these, omalizumab, an anti-IgE monoclonal antibody, has been investigated the most for its role in improving reaction thresholds and as an adjunct to oral immunotherapy for patients with IgE-mediated food allergies.[60] By binding to circulating IgE antibodies, and downregulating antigen recognizing FCεRI receptors on basophils and mast cells, omalizumab can prevent the allergic cascade and reduce the severity of allergic reactions when an individual encounters a known allergen. While not shown to be an efficacious treatment as a therapy for AD, numerous clinical trials have demonstrated the safety and efficacy of omalizumab in treating food allergies, both as an adjunct to oral immunotherapy, as well as monotherapy.[61–63] Very recently, omalizumab was approved by the FDA for individuals 1 year and older to reduce the risk of harmful reactions for those who have IgE-mediated food allergy.[64] This approval was based on results of a multicenter randomized placebo-controlled clinical trial that demonstrated that 16 weeks of treatment with omalizumab significantly improved the reaction threshold for reacting to peanut and other common food allergens.[65]

Dupilumab, a monoclonal antibody that inhibits the action of IL-4 and interleukin-13, has been at the forefront of AD treatment since its approval by the FDA for this indication in 2017. Dupilumab has also been approved for treatment of eosinophilic gastrointestinal disease in 2022. By targeting cytokines involved in the inflammatory processes associated with AD, dupilumab therapy results in significant improvements in skin symptoms, including itchiness, redness, and skin lesions, and has been found to reduce serum specific IgE to many allergenic foods.[66,67] Currently, trials are underway to evaluate its effect on food allergy, and this medication also appears to offer promise as an adjunct therapy with oral immunotherapy.[58] An understanding of overlapping immunologic mechanisms in the pathogenesis of AD and food allergy, has led to current investigation of the novel agent abrocitinib, a Janus-kinas-1 inhibitor approved for treatment of AD, for use as a potential food allergy therapeutic.[68]

While extremely promising and exciting, the use of biologic medications for the treatment of FA and AD is not without challenges. These medications can be extremely costly, and their long-term safety profiles are still being studied. However, collectively, these medications represent a potential paradigm shift in the treatment of atopic conditions, including but not limited to AD and food allergy, and will undoubtedly become more widely used therapies in the future.

SUMMARY

While there is clearly an association between AD and food allergy, the conundrum is whether there is a causal relationship between these atopic conditions. Does food allergy cause AD or does AD present a risk factor for the development of food allergy? As this article has attempted to demonstrate, the answer is not straightforward and there are still gaps in our knowledge. Children with moderate-to-severe persistent AD are at an increased risk of developing food allergy. A defective skin barrier and inflammatory milieu are likely serving as the entry point for sensitization to food allergens. However, far more children are "sensitized" to foods than are clinically allergic, and skilled allergy evaluation is crucial for establishing an accurate food allergy diagnosis. There is some danger to removing foods that are tolerated from the diet but to which a patient may be sensitized. Furthermore, delayed introduction and prolonged avoidance of allergenic foods can result in the development of IgE-mediated food allergies.

Elimination diets are not generally recommended for the treatment of atopic dermatitis, and subjecting all children with AD to unscrupulous food elimination is discouraged by expert panels and in several published guidelines. Additionally, dietary interventions, including maternal elimination diets and supplements during pregnancy, lactation, and the early infant diet, have not yet been proven to prevent or treat AD in infants and toddlers. Biologic agents used to manage many atopic conditions, are being examined in clinical trials for their therapeutic potential for both AD and food allergy. Given the evident relationship between atopic dermatitis and food allergy, these modalities are an area of continued interest and active research.

CLINICS CARE POINTS

- Typical cutaneous findings in IgE-mediated allergy are acute onset of urticaria, pruritus, angioedema, erythroderma, or flushing. AD onset and flares are not typical manifestations of food allergic reactions.

- Frequent moisturization and the use of topical anti-inflammatory medications are first-line therapies for AD, and should be optimized before considering food allergy testing in the absence of a history of acute food reactions.

- Food elimination diets are not recommended in the management of atopic dermatitis. Delayed introduction or elimination of foods from children's diets may increase the risk of food allergy development or malnutrition.

- Early introduction of allergenic foods in infancy has been shown to decrease the risk of food allergy development.

- "Sensitization" to foods (ie, positive serum IgE or skin prick testing) is far more common than clinical allergy. Skilled allergy evaluation is crucial for establishing an accurate food allergy diagnosis, particularly among children with AD.

DISCLOSURES

B. Trogen: Nothing to disclose. M. Verma: Nothing to disclose. A. Cox: Nothing to disclose. S. Sicherer: Reports royalty payments from UpToDate and from Johns Hopkins University Press; grants to his institution from the National Institute of Allergy and Infectious Diseases, United states, from Food Allergy Research and Education, United states, and from Pfizer, United states; and personal fees from the American Academy of Allergy, Asthma and Immunology as Deputy Editor of the Journal of Allergy and Clinical Immunology: In Practice, outside of the submitted work.

REFERENCES

1. Reed B, Blaiss MS. The burden of atopic dermatitis. Allergy Asthma Proc 2018;39(6):406–10.
2. Katibi OS, Cork MJ, Flohr C, et al. Moisturizer therapy in prevention of atopic dermatitis and food allergy: To use or disuse? Ann Allergy Asthma Immunol 2022;128(5):512–25.
3. Williams H, Flohr C. How epidemiology has challenged 3 prevailing concepts about atopic dermatitis. J Allergy Clin Immunol 2006;118(1):209–13.
4. Spergel JM. From atopic dermatitis to asthma: the atopic march. Ann Allergy Asthma Immunol 2010; 105(2):99–106 [quiz 7-9, 17].
5. Leung DY, Nicklas RA, Li JT, et al. Disease management of atopic dermatitis: an updated practice parameter. Joint Task Force on Practice Parameters. Ann Allergy Asthma Immunol 2004;93(3 Suppl 2): S1–21.
6. Samady W, Warren C, Kohli S, et al. The prevalence of atopic dermatitis in children with food allergy. Ann Allergy Asthma Immunol 2019;122(6):656–657 e1.
7. Singh AM, Anvari S, Hauk P, et al. Atopic dermatitis and food allergy: best practices and knowledge gaps-a work group report from the AAAAI allergic skin diseases committee and leadership institute project. J Allergy Clin Immunol Pract 2022;10(3):697–706.
8. Eller E, Kjaer HF, Host A, et al. Food allergy and food sensitization in early childhood: results from the DARC cohort. Allergy 2009;64(7):1023–9.
9. Gupta RS, Walkner MM, Greenhawt M, et al. Food allergy sensitization and presentation in siblings of food allergic children. J Allergy Clin Immunol Pract 2016;4(5):956–62.
10. Lyons SA, Clausen M, Knulst AC, et al. Prevalence of food sensitization and food allergy in children across Europe. J Allergy Clin Immunol Pract 2020;8(8): 2736–46.e9.
11. Spergel JM, Boguniewicz M, Schneider L, et al. Food allergy in infants with atopic dermatitis: limitations of food-specific IgE measurements. Pediatrics 2015;136(6):e1530–8.

12. Christensen MO, Barakji YA, Loft N, et al. Prevalence of and association between atopic dermatitis and food sensitivity, food allergy and challenge-proven food allergy: A systematic review and meta-analysis. J Eur Acad Dermatol Venereol 2023;37(5):984–1003.

13. Eigenmann PA, Calza AM. Diagnosis of IgE-mediated food allergy among Swiss children with atopic dermatitis. Pediatr Allergy Immunol 2000; 11(2):95–100.

14. Eigenmann PA, Sicherer SH, Borkowski TA, et al. Prevalence of IgE-mediated food allergy among children with atopic dermatitis. Pediatrics 1998;101(3):E8.

15. Sampson HA. The immunopathogenic role of food hypersensitivity in atopic dermatitis. Acta Derm Venereol Suppl 1992;176:34–7.

16. Gupta RS, Warren CM, Smith BM, et al. The public health impact of parent-reported childhood food allergies in the United States. Pediatrics 2018;142(6).

17. Peters RL, Koplin JJ, Gurrin LC, et al. The prevalence of food allergy and other allergic diseases in early childhood in a population-based study: Health-Nuts age 4-year follow-up. J Allergy Clin Immunol 2017;140(1):145–53.e8.

18. Hill DJ, Hosking CS, de Benedictis FM, et al. Confirmation of the association between high levels of immunoglobulin E food sensitization and eczema in infancy: an international study. Clin Exp Allergy 2008;38(1):161–8.

19. Lack G, Fox D, Northstone K, et al. Factors associated with the development of peanut allergy in childhood. N Engl J Med 2003;348(11):977–85.

20. Langan SM, Irvine AD, Weidinger S. Atopic dermatitis. Lancet 2020;396(10247):345–60.

21. Fukiwake N, Furusyo N, Takeoka H, et al. Association factors for atopic dermatitis in nursery school children in Ishigaki islands - Kyushu University Ishigaki Atopic Dermatitis Study (KIDS). Eur J Dermatol 2008;18(5):571–4.

22. Johansson EK, Bergstrom A, Kull I, et al. IgE sensitization in relation to preschool eczema and filaggrin mutation. J Allergy Clin Immunol 2017;140(6): 1572–1579 e5.

23. Papapostolou N, Xepapadaki P, Gregoriou S, et al. Atopic dermatitis and food allergy: a complex interplay what we know and what we would like to learn. J Clin Med 2022;11(14).

24. Weidinger S, Beck LA, Bieber T, et al. Atopic dermatitis. Nat Rev Dis Prim 2018;4(1):1.

25. Graves PE, Kabesch M, Halonen M, et al. A cluster of seven tightly linked polymorphisms in the IL-13 gene is associated with total serum IgE levels in three populations of white children. J Allergy Clin Immunol 2000;105(3):506–13.

26. Zitnik SE, Ruschendorf F, Muller S, et al. IL13 variants are associated with total serum IgE and early sensitization to food allergens in children with atopic dermatitis. Pediatr Allergy Immunol 2009;20(6):551–5.

27. Palmer CN, Irvine AD, Terron-Kwiatkowski A, et al. Common loss-of-function variants of the epidermal barrier protein filaggrin are a major predisposing factor for atopic dermatitis. Nat Genet 2006;38(4):441–6.

28. Astolfi A, Cipriani F, Messelodi D, et al. Filaggrin loss-of-function mutations are risk factors for severe food allergy in children with atopic dermatitis. J Clin Med 2021;10(2).

29. Asai Y, Greenwood C, Hull PR, et al. Filaggrin gene mutation associations with peanut allergy persist despite variations in peanut allergy diagnostic criteria or asthma status. J Allergy Clin Immunol 2013;132(1):239–42.

30. Brough HA, Liu AH, Sicherer S, et al. Atopic dermatitis increases the effect of exposure to peanut antigen in dust on peanut sensitization and likely peanut allergy. J Allergy Clin Immunol 2015;135(1):164–70.

31. Ashley SE, Tan HT, Vuillermin P, et al. The skin barrier function gene SPINK5 is associated with challenge-proven IgE-mediated food allergy in infants. Allergy 2017;72(9):1356–64.

32. Miyaji Y, Yang L, Yamamoto-Hanada K, et al. Earlier aggressive treatment to shorten the duration of eczema in infants resulted in fewer food allergies at 2 years of age. J Allergy Clin Immunol Pract 2020;8(5):1721–1724 e6.

33. Wood RA, Camargo CA Jr, Lieberman P, et al. Anaphylaxis in America: the prevalence and characteristics of anaphylaxis in the United States. J Allergy Clin Immunol 2014;133(2):461–7.

34. Sicherer SH, Sampson HA. Food hypersensitivity and atopic dermatitis: pathophysiology, epidemiology, diagnosis, and management. J Allergy Clin Immunol 1999;104(3 Pt 2):S114–22.

35. Roerdink EM, Flokstra-de Blok BM, Blok JL, et al. Association of food allergy and atopic dermatitis exacerbations. Ann Allergy Asthma Immunol 2016; 116(4):334–8.

36. Sampson HA, McCaskill CC. Food hypersensitivity and atopic dermatitis: evaluation of 113 patients. J Pediatr 1985;107(5):669–75.

37. Burks AW, Mallory SB, Williams LW, et al. Atopic dermatitis: clinical relevance of food hypersensitivity reactions. J Pediatr 1988;113(3):447–51.

38. Breuer K, Wulf A, Constien A, et al. Birch pollen-related food as a provocation factor of allergic symptoms in children with atopic eczema/dermatitis syndrome. Allergy 2004;59(9):988–94.

39. Chu DK, Schneider L, Asiniwasis RN, et al. Atopic dermatitis (eczema) guidelines: 2023 American Academy of Allergy, Asthma and Immunology/American College of Allergy, Asthma and Immunology Joint Task Force on Practice Parameters GRADE- and Institute of Medicine-based recommendations. Ann Allergy Asthma Immunol 2023;132(3):274–312.

40. Greer FR, Sicherer SH, Burks AW, et al. Immunology. The effects of early nutritional interventions on the development of atopic disease in infants and

children: the role of maternal dietary restriction, breastfeeding, hydrolyzed formulas, and timing of introduction of allergenic complementary foods. Pediatrics 2019;143(4).

41. Greer FR, Sicherer SH, Burks AW. American Academy of Pediatrics Committee on N, American Academy of Pediatrics Section on A, Immunology. Effects of early nutritional interventions on the development of atopic disease in infants and children: the role of maternal dietary restriction, breastfeeding, timing of introduction of complementary foods, and hydrolyzed formulas. Pediatrics 2008;121(1):183–91.

42. Gdalevich M, Mimouni D, David M, et al. Breastfeeding and the onset of atopic dermatitis in childhood: A systematic review and meta-analysis of prospective studies. J Am Acad Dermatol 2001;45(4):520–7.

43. Lodge CJ, Tan DJ, Lau MX, et al. Breastfeeding and asthma and allergies: a systematic review and meta-analysis. Acta Paediatr 2015;104(467):38–53.

44. Kramer MS, Kakuma R. Optimal duration of exclusive breastfeeding. Cochrane Database Syst Rev 2012;2012(8):CD003517.

45. Osborn DA, Sinn J. Soy formula for prevention of allergy and food intolerance in infants. Cochrane Database Syst Rev 2006;2006(4):CD003741.

46. Khan A, Adalsteinsson J, Whitaker-Worth DL. Atopic dermatitis and nutrition. Clin Dermatol 2022;40(2):135–44.

47. Kim MJ, Kim SN, Lee YW, et al. Vitamin D status and efficacy of Vitamin D supplementation in atopic dermatitis: a systematic review and meta-analysis. Nutrients 2016;8(12).

48. Makrgeorgou A, Leonardi-Bee J, Bath-Hextall FJ, et al. Probiotics for treating eczema. Cochrane Database Syst Rev 2018;11(11):Cd006135.

49. Zhao M, Shen C, Ma L. Treatment efficacy of probiotics on atopic dermatitis, zooming in on infants: a systematic review and meta-analysis. Int J Dermatol 2018;57(6):635–41.

50. Perkin MR, Logan K, Marrs T, et al. Association of frequent moisturizer use in early infancy with the development of food allergy. J Allergy Clin Immunol 2021;147(3):967–976 e1.

51. Oykhman P, Dookie J, Al-Rammahy H, et al. Dietary elimination for the treatment of atopic dermatitis: a systematic review and meta-analysis. J Allergy Clin Immunol Pract 2022;10(10):2657–66.e8.

52. Du Toit G, Roberts G, Sayre PH, et al. Randomized trial of peanut consumption in infants at risk for peanut allergy. N Engl J Med 2015;372(9):803–13.

53. Chang A, Robison R, Cai M, et al. Natural history of food-triggered atopic dermatitis and development of immediate reactions in children. J Allergy Clin Immunol Pract 2016;4(2):229–236 e1.

54. Trogen B, Jacobs S, Nowak-Wegrzyn A. Early introduction of allergenic foods and the prevention of food allergy. Nutrients 2022;14(13).

55. Sariachvili M, Droste J, Dom S, et al. Early exposure to solid foods and the development of eczema in children up to 4 years of age. Pediatr Allergy Immunol 2010;21(1 Pt 1):74–81.

56. Tromp II, Kiefte-de Jong JC, Lebon A, et al. The introduction of allergenic foods and the development of reported wheezing and eczema in childhood: the Generation R study. Arch Pediatr Adolesc Med 2011;165(10):933–8.

57. Zutavern A, Brockow I, Schaaf B, et al. Timing of solid food introduction in relation to eczema, asthma, allergic rhinitis, and food and inhalant sensitization at the age of 6 years: results from the prospective birth cohort study LISA. Pediatrics 2008;121(1):e44–52.

58. Sindher SB, Fiocchi A, Zuberbier T, et al. The role of biologics in the treatment of food allergy. J Allergy Clin Immunol Pract 2023;12(3):562–8.

59. Cook-Mills JM, Emmerson LN. Epithelial barrier regulation, antigen sampling, and food allergy. J Allergy Clin Immunol 2022;150(3):493–502.

60. Zuberbier T, Wood RA, Bindslev-Jensen C, et al. Omalizumab in IgE-mediated food allergy: a systematic review and meta-analysis. J Allergy Clin Immunol Pract 2023;11(4):1134–46.

61. Yee CSK, Albuhairi S, Noh E, et al. Long-term outcome of peanut oral immunotherapy facilitated initially by omalizumab. J Allergy Clin Immunol Pract 2019;7(2):451–461 e7.

62. MacGinnitie AJ, Rachid R, Gragg H, et al. Omalizumab facilitates rapid oral desensitization for peanut allergy. J Allergy Clin Immunol 2017;139(3):873–881 e8.

63. Martorell-Calatayud C, Michavila-Gomez A, Martorell-Aragones A, et al. Anti-IgE-assisted desensitization to egg and cow's milk in patients refractory to conventional oral immunotherapy. Pediatr Allergy Immunol 2016;27(5):544–6.

64. FDA approves omalizumab for food allergies. Available at: https://www.fda.gov/news-events/press-announcements/fda-approves-first-medication-help-reduce-allergic-reactions-multiple-foods-after-accidental.

65. Wood RA, Togias A, Sicherer SH, et al. Omalizumab for the Treatment of multiple food allergies. N Engl J Med 2024;390(10):889–99.

66. Guttman-Yassky E, Bissonnette R, Ungar B, et al. Dupilumab progressively improves systemic and cutaneous abnormalities in patients with atopic dermatitis. J Allergy Clin Immunol 2019;143(1):155–72.

67. Spekhorst LS, van der Rijst LP, de Graaf M, et al. Dupilumab has a profound effect on specific-IgE levels of several food allergens in atopic dermatitis patients. Allergy 2023;78(3):875–8.

68. Berin MC. Targeting type 2 immunity and the future of food allergy treatment. J Exp Med 2023;220(4).

Patient Burden of Atopic Dermatitis and Opportunities for Real-World Self-Monitoring

Wendy Smith Begolka, MBS[a],*, Jessica K. Johnson, MPH[a],
Isabelle J. Thibau, MPH[a]

KEYWORDS

- Atopic dermatitis ● Eczema ● Patient ● Burden ● Symptoms ● Quality of life ● Disease monitoring

KEY POINTS

- Patient burden of disease in atopic dermatitis (AD) is significant, dynamic, and heterogeneous.
- While itch, skin erythema, and sleep disruption are the most problematic patient-reported AD symptoms, the impact of disease affects emotional, psychological, social, lifestyle, work/school, and financial well-being.
- Patient (or caregiver) self-monitoring of AD has the potential to enhance disease management and allow patients to be more active partners in their care and treatment.
- Digital tools for patient self-monitoring are available to support tracking specific AD symptoms and other aspects of disease burden.

INTRODUCTION

Atopic dermatitis (AD) is a chronic, relapsing, inflammatory skin disease affecting over 31 million individuals in the United States alone, with an onset that occurs at any age.[1–3] Globally, AD is a leading contributor to disease-related disability, ranking 15th among all nonfatal diseases, and first among skin diseases.[4] This rank stems from the growing range of negative impacts on health, quality of life (QoL), and well-being for affected individuals. AD is notable for its clinical complexity, with variable disease trajectory, intensity, presentation, and persistence.[5] The lived experience burden of AD is equally complex and goes far beyond skin-related considerations (**Fig. 1**). A survey of 1065 adult patients indicated the disease journey is multidimensional, heterogeneous, and without any single aspect driving the overall AD burden.[6]

Understanding the current and cumulative lifetime patient burden of AD across all severities, including those with milder or more limited disease, is important to facilitate holistic AD care. Further, as AD burdens include those visible and unseen, patient-reported contributions to periodic assessments of health and QoL status are essential to fully appreciate the constellation of impacts, and their variation between patients. Herein, we discuss the myriad contributors to AD patient burden and the opportunity to engage patients via self-monitoring of ongoing impact.

HOLISTIC BURDEN OF ATOPIC DERMATITIS

AD presents many dynamic physical burdens for affected individuals primarily due to its unpredictable disease course, and presence or recurrence of inadequately controlled symptoms.[7,8] Patients

[a] National Eczema Association, 505 San Marin Drive, #B300, Novato, CA 94945, USA
* Corresponding author. 505 San Marin Drive, #B300 Novato, CA 94945
E-mail address: wendy@nationaleczema.org

Dermatol Clin 42 (2024) 537–548
https://doi.org/10.1016/j.det.2024.04.007

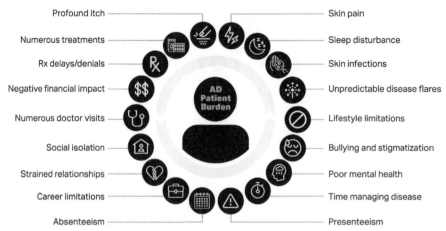

Profound itch — Skin pain
Numerous treatments — Sleep disturbance
Rx delays/denials — Skin infections
Negative financial impact — Unpredictable disease flares
Numerous doctor visits — Lifestyle limitations
Social isolation — Bullying and stigmatization
Strained relationships — Poor mental health
Career limitations — Time managing disease
Absenteeism — Presenteeism

Fig. 1. Holistic patient-reported burden of atopic dermatitis (AD).

navigate waxing and waning disease severity, with some never achieving clear/almost clear skin and variations in the amount and location of skin involvement and the frequency and intensity of disease flares. Nearly two-thirds of participants (64%) in the 2019 More Than Skin Deep (MTSD) survey indicated more or different body areas affected by AD since initial diagnosis, with only 33% indicating that flare frequency has lessened over time.[9] A 2006 survey of adults with AD reported a yearly average of 9 flare episodes with an average duration of 15 days each, with flare severity and duration increasing with disease severity.[10] A prospective study of US children with AD indicated that greater than 80% have ongoing symptoms with little relief, and only 50% have 1 or more disease-free periods by age 20.[11]

Itch is the most prevalent and problematic symptom for patients regardless of disease severity.[9,12,13] The number of daily itch episodes has been reported to range from 1 to greater than 10, with nearly two-thirds of patients having at least 5.[14] A recent prospective study demonstrated significant longitudinal variation in patient-reported itch scores, with few achieving complete itch remission.[15] Nocturnal scratching is a further challenge for AD patients, leading to sleep disruption and waking to bleeding scratch marks, stained sheets and clothing.[9] Parents of children with AD often co-sleep to attempt to alleviate itch-related burdens, creating additional familial impacts.[16] The collective negative impact of persistent itch on patient's lives is substantial, resulting in a relational effect on additional negative AD symptoms and outcomes (**Fig. 2**). Patients attribute significant negative emotional sentiment to itch, using words such as 'nightmarish," "torture," and "uncontrollable."[9]

Frequent dry, sensitive skin alongside other skin issues (eg, inflammation, roughness, oozing, flaking, pigmentation changes, and skin pain) also negatively affects patients, both as symptoms as well as on impact to QoL, particularly for clothing choices and social activities.[9,12,17] Damaged and/ or compromised skin also presents an increased risk for infections and furthers the disease burden.

Sleep disturbance is prevalent among both AD patients and caregivers, ranking among the top 3 most burdensome symptoms, often more so for caregivers than adult patients.[9,18] Patients experience difficulty falling asleep and staying asleep, leading to poor overall sleep quality and insomnia.[19,20] Sixty percent of caregivers have reported waking 2 or more times per night to attend to their child.[21] Long-term sleep deprivation can lead to poor overall physical health and further negative effects for patients and caregivers resulting in daytime fatigue and sleepiness; changes in mood and attention; and challenges with work/ school presenteeism and productivity.[22]

Mental Health

AD patients often experience psychological distress, including anxiety, depression, and in some cases suicidality.[9,23–26] A recent survey by the National Eczema Association (NEA) of 1496 AD patients and caregivers found 71% of respondents reported negative mental health from their AD in the past 12 months and 1 in 4 reported mental health symptoms for greater than 10 days in the past month, especially those with more severe AD.[27]

The contributors to poor mental health in AD are numerous. Undesirable appearance and condition of the skin affects patient self-image and confidence, resulting in feelings of embarrassment,

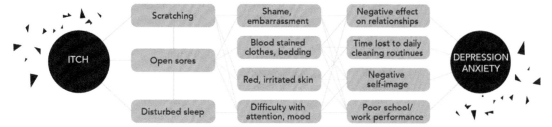

Fig. 2. The effects of itch on other symptoms and life impacts. (*Reprinted from* McCleary KK. More Than Skin Deep "Voice of the Patient" Report. 2020. March 2020. http://www.morethanskindeep-eczema.org/uploads/1/2/5/3/125377765/mtsd_report_-_digital_file.pdf. Under a Creative Commons Attribution 4.0 International License.)

shame, and isolation.[9,10,22] Nearly 40% of school-aged children and teens with AD have experienced appearance-based bullying or stigmatization because of their AD.[28,29] The potential for and reoccurrence of flares contribute to considerable patient anxiety and negative emotional sentiment,[10,30] making reduced flares the second-most important treatment outcome for AD patients.[9] Patients and caregivers also harbor concerns related to limited treatment efficacy, and the fear of long-term treatment side effects and comorbidities.[31] Caregivers also experience feelings of guilt, exhaustion, frustration, and helplessness.[21] Collectively, AD's negative impact on mental health ranks greater than that for patients with other chronic conditions such as heart disease and diabetes, leading a recent review to suggest that the psychological burden of AD can be as burdensome to manage as physical symptoms.[12,32]

Quality of Life

A US population-based survey reported adults with AD were more likely to rate their overall health as 'only fair'/'poor,' and satisfaction with life as 'somewhat dissatisfied'/'very dissatisfied,' compared to those unaffected by AD.[12] When asked about the overall burden of AD in the past month, 51% of MTSD survey participants reported a high/significant impact on their QoL.[6] Everyday activities can be challenging for AD patients. In a study of 602 adult patients with AD, over half reported lifestyle limitations, 40% avoided social interactions due to their appearance, and 43% stated AD had a negative impact on their social activities.[12] Individuals with AD on more visible areas such as the head/neck and hands have been reported to experience greater effects on QoL.[33]

AD can impact work and school attendance and have long-term impacts on career and job choices.[22,34] In a study of 200 children with AD and psoriasis, 62.5% with AD missed greater than 1 day of school and 3.6% missed 15 or more days

due to their disease.[35] Parents of children with AD are more likely to miss work days than other parents, and report long and repeated periods of time taken off of work due to AD care appointments.[9,35] Caregivers of children with AD can also find it difficult to have careers or jobs where they work outside of the home due to the need to provide a standard of care for their child.[9]

The physical burden of AD, coupled with the psychological impact, can make it more challenging for AD patients to create and sustain interpersonal relationships. Patients and caregivers reported damage to clothing, furnishings, and bedding from topical treatments, flaking skin, and blood to have a negative impact on their relationships.[9] As patients enter adulthood, new AD burdens arise such as negative effects on sexual health and strained marital and family relationships.[36,37] Partners of patients with AD also experience challenges and adjustments to their daily activities.[36]

Treatment and Management Burden

AD is a time-consuming and complex condition to manage. US children and adults with AD have more outpatient office and emergency department visits, and hospital admissions with prolonged hospitalizations compared to those without AD.[38] Management regimens include multiple prescription and non-prescription products and medications, trigger avoidance, lifestyle modifications, and supportive care items that often change over time.[39] Polypharmacy is common for AD with 57.5% of recent adult AD survey respondents (n = 1118) reporting use of greater than 3 prescription treatments in the past year.[40] Prescription numbers increase with the presence of AD comorbid conditions.[41] Increased time spent managing symptoms has been shown to have a strong association with patient-reported disease burden.[6] The 1508 adult MTSD survey respondents reported nearly 50% spend greater than 5 h/wk managing symptoms, with 23% spending greater than 11 h/wk.[9]

Table 1 Harmonizing outcome measures for eczema core outcome set for clinical practice		
Instrument Name	Construct	Description
Patient Oriented Scoring for Atopic Dermatitis (PO-SCORAD) index	Disease severity	8-item, PRO for monitoring symptom intensity, itch, and sleeplessness over the past 48 h (Stalder, 2011)
Patient Oriented Eczema Measure	Disease severity	7-item, PRO for monitoring atopic eczema severity over the past week (Charman, 2004)
Peak 24-h Numeric Rating Scale (NRS) itch	Itch severity	Single-item, PRO for monitoring itch severity in the past 24 h (Yosipovitch, 2019)
Average 1-wk NRS-itch (Patient-Reported Outcomes Information System (PROMIS) Itch Questionnaire)	Itch severity	Single-item, PRO for monitoring itch severity over the past week (Silverberg, Patel, et al, 2020)
Peak 1-wk NRS-itch (PROMIS Itch Questionnaire)	Itch severity	Single-item, for monitoring itch severity over the past week (Silverberg, Patel, et al, 2020)
Recap of Atopic Eczema (RECAP)	Disease control	7-item, PRO for monitoring eczema control over the past week (Howells, 2019)
Atopic Dermatitis Control Tool (ADCT)	Disease control	6-item, PRO for monitoring AD control over the past week (Parisier, 2019)

Abbreviations: AD, atopic dermatitis; PRO, patient-reported outcome.

From Leshem YA, Chalmers JR, Apfelbacher C, et al. Measuring atopic eczema symptoms in clinical practice: The first consensus statement from the Harmonising Outcome Measures for Eczema in clinical practice initiative. J Am Acad Dermatol. May 2020;82(5):1181-1186. https://doi.org/10.1016/j.jaad.2019.12.055.

AD is also associated with considerable financial burden. The median annual patient-reported out-of-pocket (OOP) expense has been recently estimated at $600, with 42% of study respondents spending more than $1000/y, and 9% spending more than $5000/y[39] In 2015, annual direct costs of AD were estimated to exceed $5.3 billion, with over $600 million due to lost productivity from affected individuals and caregivers.[42] The harmful financial impact of AD is compounded by frequent polypharmacy and insurance coverage issues for medications.[41,43] Delays and denials for both established and recently approved AD therapies are common, leading to delayed and unfilled prescriptions increasing patient burden, and increased OOP for prescriptions not covered by insurance.[39] Recent NEA survey results suggest 48% of adult AD respondents experienced at least 1 insurance delay or denial for their AD prescriptions in the past year, with only half of respondents indicating they would know what to do if they experienced challenges with insurance prescription coverage.[44]

REAL-WORLD PATIENT SELF-MONITORING

Self-management is defined as steps individuals undertake to live with their condition, including confidence to navigate medical and emotional management considerations.[45] Examples of self-management include awareness of symptoms and triggers, responding to changes in health with appropriate actions, making lifestyle changes, adhering to therapies, and making office visits for clinical care.[45] Self-monitoring is a key component of self-management, where tracking and recording of symptoms or other aspects of health can support adjustment of behaviors, lifestyle, and treatments in response to recorded data either independently or in consultation with a health care provider (HCP).[46–48]

Self-monitoring is frequently done for other chronic diseases, such as high blood pressure, diabetes, and asthma, and is being explored for many others that, like AD, share an inherent variability for and between individuals over time.[49]

Patient Education via Self-Monitoring

Self-monitoring as a component of self-management is not new to AD patients. Journaling, taking photos, tracking flares, and making lists to note exposures to potential triggers has been a mainstay in patient self-monitoring to try to understand their disease through documenting trends and issues of concern.[9]

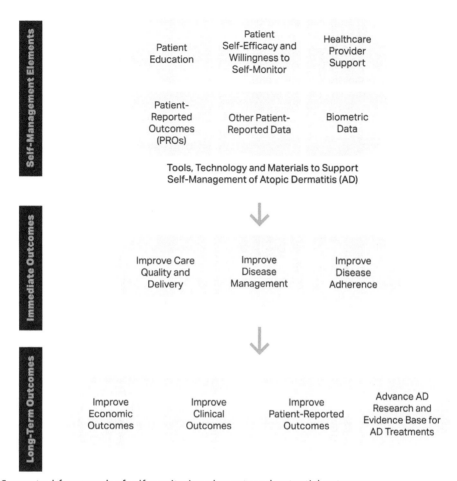

Fig. 3. Conceptual framework of self-monitoring elements and potential outcomes.

At a minimum, self-monitoring by AD patients serves as a form of patient education. Through tracking and recording various aspects of health status, patients gain awareness and confidence in recognizing symptoms, signs, and triggers, which enables a growing understanding of their disease course and the appropriate use of treatments.[50] Further, it provides patients with a mechanism to turn qualitative assessments into something more tangible and quantifiable, and less susceptible to recall bias.

Self-Monitoring to Enhance Care

As most of an individual's time is not spent with their HCP, and daily management decisions and disease experiences occur outside of health care settings, there is opportunity to foster patient engagement in managing their condition to achieve desired outcomes. The use of information from patient self-monitoring to inform changes in AD disease management has not been studied to date but has the potential to provide new insights into the real-world patient experience, and improvements or worsening of disease burden in-between HCP visits. This potential coincides with the increased recognition of the value of patient-reported outcomes (PROs) as part of AD care.[51]

The Harmonizing Outcome Measures for Eczema (HOME) initiative has prioritized instruments for inclusion in a clinical practice set (Table 1), covering PROs for symptoms and control, with work ongoing to align on patient global assessment, clinician-reported signs, and eczema-specific QoL.[52] By extension, the HOME recommendations can serve as a guide and starting point for how patient self-monitoring could complement PROs collection at HCP visits and provide a more comprehensive and holistic picture of the disease. The selection of specific items and the frequency of patient self-monitoring has also not been studied, albeit something that could be determined collaboratively

Table 2
Selection of digital tools available to atopic dermatitis patients in the United States to self-monitor their disease and the components of self-monitoring available at no added cost

Tool Name	Developer	Uniform Resource Locator	Tool Type	Patient-Reported Outcome Collection Construct (Validated Instrument)	Other Patient-Reported Data	Data Interpretation	Shared Decision-Making	Patient Education
Atopic App	Avanta JSC	https://atopicapp.com/	Mobile app	Disease severity/quality of life (POEM); stress	Treatments taken; photos; environmental exposures; diet	PRO trends graph; environmental exposures trends graph; PRO score interpretation; artificial intelligence disease severity tool; treatment adherence report	Action plan	App orientation/tooltips; educational articles.
DLQI App	Cardiff University	https://play.google.com/store/apps/details?id=uk.ac.cardiff.dlqi&hl=en_US&gl=US	Mobile app	Quality of life (DLQI)	n/a	PRO score interpretation	n/a	n/a
Eczema App Nia	Nia Health Gmbh	https://www.nia-medtech.com/	Mobile app	Disease severity (PO-SCORAD); Quality of life (DLQI); flares	Treatments taken; photos; environmental exposures; diet	PRO trends graph (up to 1 month); PRO score interpretation	n/a	App orientation/tooltips
Eczema Care+	Pierre Fabre Eczema Association	https://play.google.com/store/apps/details?id=com.eczema foundation.eczemacareplus	Mobile app	Disease severity (PO-SCORAD); quality of life (DLQI)	Photos; environmental exposures	PRO trends graph; artificial intelligence disease severity tool	Action plan; preparatory questions for upcoming appointment; corticosteroid knowledge	App orientation/tooltips; educational articles/videos

EczemaLess	Polyfins Technology	https://eczemaless.com/	Mobile app	Disease severity/quality of life (POEM); itch (NRS)	Treatments taken; environmental exposures; diet	PRO trends graph; PRO score interpretation; artificial intelligence disease severity tool	n/a	n/a
Eczema Manager for Atopic Dermatitis	At Point of Care, LLC	https://apps.apple.com/us/app/eczema-manager/id1364065458	Mobile app	Global health; pain (NRS); itch; Disease severity/quality of life (POEM); mental health (PHQ-4); sleep (Fatigue SF6a, Sleep disturbance SF4a)	Treatments taken; photos; physical activity	PRO trends graph	Appointment checklist	App orientation/tooltips; educational articles/videos
EczemaWise	National Eczema Association (NEA)	https://www.eczemawise.org/	Mobile app and Web platform	Disease severity (PO-SCORAD); itch (NRS); sleep (NRS); pain (NRS); stress (NRS); quality of life (Skindex Mini[60]); quality of life (DLQI); self-report preparedness for health visits	Treatments taken; photos; environmental exposures; diet;	PRO trends graph; daily tracking data; PRO score interpretation; year-over-year progress report	Preparatory questions for upcoming appointment; self-reported treatment considerations	App orientation/tooltips; treatment decision aid; educational articles/videos
My Eczema Tracker	The University of Nottingham	https://www.nottingham.ac.uk/research/groups/cebd/resources/my-eczema-tracker-app.aspx	Mobile app	Disease severity/quality of life (POEM); eczema control (RECAP)	n/a	PRO trends graph; PRO score interpretation	n/a	n/a

(continued on next page)

Table 2
(continued)

Tool Name	Developer	Uniform Resource Locator	Tool Type	Patient-Reported Outcome Collection Construct (Validated Instrument)	Other Patient-Reported Data	Data Interpretation	Shared Decision-Making	Patient Education
My Derm	Ampersand Health Limited	https://ampersandhealth.co.uk/myderm/	Mobile app	Pain; sleep; itch; mood; exercise; quality of life (DLQI)	n/a	PRO trends graph;	n/a	App orientation/tooltips; educational articles/videos
MySkinHealth - Fontus Health Eczema	Fontus Health	https://www.myskinhealth.org/	Mobile app	Disease severity/quality of life (POEM); disease severity (EASI)	Photos	PRO trends graph; PRO score interpretation	Action plan	Educational articles/videos
NALA	NALA	https://nala.care/en/the-app/	Mobile app	Disease severity (PO-SCORAD); itch; stress; sleep; emotional health; quality of life (DLQI)	Treatments taken; photos; environmental exposures; diet; physical activity	PRO score interpretation	n/a	n/a
Sidekick Health	Sidekick Health AB	https://sidekicktherapeutics.com/ca-ad/	Mobile app	Itch; sleep; stress; energy; skin health	Photos; diet; physical activity	n/a	n/a	App orientation/tooltips; educational articles/videos

mHealth Apps available as of January 2024 in the Apple or Google Play Stores for download and account creation.

Abbreviations: AD, atopic dermatitis; DLQI, dermatology life quality index; EASI, eczema area and severity index; Fatigue SF6a, fatigue short form 6a; NRS, numeric rating scale; PHQ-4, patient health questionnaire-4; POEM, patient-oriented eczema measure; PO-SCORAD, patient-oriented scoring for atopic dermatitis; PRO, patient-reported outcome; Sleep Disturbance SF4a, sleep disturbance short form 4a.

between patients and their HCP based on treatment goals and existing burden as part of ongoing shared decision-making (SDM).

Current data suggest AD patients are generally willing to engage in self-monitoring as part of their disease management, and desire an opportunity to use this information to engage in a patient-tailored approach to care.[53–55] A recent qualitative study with adult AD patients identified the need for an increased role of patients in determining physical and emotional impact of disease alongside discussion of needs and preferences in AD care.[56]

Fig. 3 presents a conceptual framework of elements of AD self-monitoring and potential downstream effects. Future studies should explore the ability of patient-driven information to support patient education, SDM, treatment adherence, clinical outcomes and PROs, and patient satisfaction, while minimizing health care costs, insurance challenges, and overall disease burden for AD. Resources and approaches to help guide patients and HCPs in the effective use of self-monitoring tools are also needed in order to avoid additional burden.

Digital Tools for Patient Self-Monitoring

Patient diaries are a simple form of journaling and tracking health; however, they are not standardized and do not generally include quantitative measures. In the past decade, there has been a marked increase in the development and public acceptance of various mobile health applications (mHealth apps). A 2018 systematic assessment of patient-facing AD mHealth apps revealed large variances in the quality and comprehensiveness of educational information and tracking capabilities and identified opportunities for improvement to support evidence-based self-monitoring.[57] Since 2018, more AD mHealth apps have entered the space to attempt to address these gaps. Currently, 12 digital tools are now available for patients in the United States to support self-monitoring (**Table 2**); additional apps are available to patients outside the United States. These US-facing apps have been developed by an eczema patient advocacy organization (NEA), academic institutions, pharmaceutical and health-related companies, and start-up technology corporations. Collectively, they vary in their involvement of AD patients/caregivers and HCPs in app development, use of validated PROs for AD such as those recommended by HOME, provision of educational information, support of SDM, and use of artificial intelligence. While the prevalence of digital tools for AD continues to increase, only 3 have data available

related to their use for patient self-monitoring, education, or care management.[53,55,58]

Other tools including wearable technologies that collect biometric data relevant to AD (eg, sleep quality, itch, nocturnal scratching, transepidermal water loss), and often accompanied by a mobile app are also in development.[59,60] As some of these tools are not yet widely available outside of research settings, or are used primarily for general fitness or health and wellness (eg, watches, rings, bands), their use as a component of AD self-monitoring is yet to be determined.

SUMMARY

The patient burden of AD is multidimensional and heterogeneous, involving impacts that are visible and unseen. A holistic and real-world understanding of disease burden is only possible with insights directly from patients. Self-monitoring of AD burdensome symptoms and QoL by patients has the potential to be a valuable component of overall disease management and provide additional information about improvements or worsening in health and well-being that can complement data collected in the health care setting. Journaling approaches as well as digital tools can be used to support patient self-monitoring. HCPs and patients have an opportunity to work together to identify aspects of self-monitoring that would be the most helpful to support treatment goals and alleviation of patient burden.

CLINICS CARE POINTS

- The patient burden of AD is complex and can vary from patient to patient, or for the same person over time regarding the most burdensome aspects of disease and treatment.

- A holistic appreciation of patient burden can be accomplished with input from patients through use of PROs and/or information from patient self-monitoring.

- Ongoing discussion between patients and HCPs can facilitate alignment on aspects of disease burden that would benefit from periodic assessment in the clinic and real-world settings.

DISCLOSURES

W. Smith Begolka, J.K. Johnson, and I.J. Thibau are salaried employees of the NEA. W. Smith Begolka has received advisory board honoraria from Sanofi, Amgen, and Pfizer and research grants from Pfizer, United States.

REFERENCES

1. Hanifin JM, Reed ML, Eczema P, et al. A population-based survey of eczema prevalence in the United States. Dermatitis 2007;18(2):82–91.

2. Shaw TE, Currie GP, Koudelka CW, et al. Eczema prevalence in the United States: data from the 2003 National Survey of Children's Health. J Invest Dermatol 2011;131(1):67–73.

3. Lee HH, Patel KR, Singam V, et al. A systematic review and meta-analysis of the prevalence and phenotype of adult-onset atopic dermatitis. J Am Acad Dermatol 2019;80(6):1526–1532 e7.

4. Laughter MR, Maymone MBC, Mashayekhi S, et al. The global burden of atopic dermatitis: lessons from the Global Burden of Disease Study 1990-2017. Br J Dermatol 2021;184(2):304–9.

5. Chovatiya R, Silverberg JI. Evaluating the longitudinal course of atopic dermatitis: A review of the literature. J Am Acad Dermatol 2022;87(3):688–9.

6. Elsawi R, Dainty K, Smith Begolka W, et al. The multidimensional burden of atopic dermatitis among adults: results from a large national survey. JAMA Dermatol 2022;158(8):887–92.

7. Simpson EL, Guttman-Yassky E, Margolis DJ, et al. Association of inadequately controlled disease and disease severity with patient-reported disease burden in adults with atopic dermatitis. JAMA Dermatol 2018;154(8):903–12.

8. Wei W, Anderson P, Gadkari A, et al. Extent and consequences of inadequate disease control among adults with a history of moderate to severe atopic dermatitis. J Dermatol 2018;45(2):150–7.

9. McCleary K.K., More than skin deep "voice of the patient" report, Available at: http://www.morethanskindeep-eczema.org/uploads/1/2/5/3/125377765/mtsd_report_-_digital_file.pdf, 2020. Accessed December 1, 2023.

10. Zuberbier T, Orlow SJ, Paller AS, et al. Patient perspectives on the management of atopic dermatitis. J Allergy Clin Immunol 2006;118(1):226–32.

11. Margolis JS, Abuabara K, Bilker W, et al. Persistence of mild to moderate atopic dermatitis. JAMA Dermatol 2014;150(6):593–600.

12. Silverberg JI, Gelfand JM, Margolis DJ, et al. Patient burden and quality of life in atopic dermatitis in US adults: A population-based cross-sectional study. Ann Allergy Asthma Immunol 2018;121(3):340–7.

13. Bacci E, Rentz A, Correll J, et al. Patient-reported disease burden and unmet therapeutic needs in atopic dermatitis. J Drugs Dermatol 2021;20(11):1222–30.

14. Dawn A, Papoiu AD, Chan YH, et al. Itch characteristics in atopic dermatitis: results of a web-based questionnaire. Br J Dermatol 2009;160(3):642–4.

15. Hong MR, Lei D, Yousaf M, et al. A real-world study of the longitudinal course of adult atopic dermatitis severity in clinical practice. Ann Allergy Asthma Immunol 2020;125(6):686–692 e3.

16. Chamlin SL, Mattson CL, Frieden IJ, et al. The price of pruritus: sleep disturbance and cosleeping in atopic dermatitis. Arch Pediatr Adolesc Med 2005;159(8):745–50.

17. Vakharia PP, Chopra R, Sacotte R, et al. Burden of skin pain in atopic dermatitis. Ann Allergy Asthma Immunol 2017;119(6):548–552 e3.

18. Ramirez FD, Chen S, Langan SM, et al. Assessment of sleep disturbances and exhaustion in mothers of children with atopic dermatitis. JAMA Dermatol 2019;155(5):556–63.

19. Silverberg JI, Chiesa-Fuxench Z, Margolis D, et al. Epidemiology and burden of sleep disturbances in atopic dermatitis in US Adults. Dermatitis Nov-01 2022;33(6S):S104–13.

20. Li JC, Fishbein A, Singam V, et al. Sleep disturbance and sleep-related impairment in adults with atopic dermatitis: a cross-sectional study. Dermatitis Sep-2018;29(5):270–7.

21. Capozza K, Gadd H, Kelley K, et al. Insights from caregivers on the impact of pediatric atopic dermatitis on families: "i'm tired, overwhelmed, and feel like i'm failing as a mother". Dermatitis May/2020;31(3):223–7.

22. Bacci ED, Correll JR, Pierce EJ, et al. Burden of adult atopic dermatitis and unmet needs with existing therapies. J Dermatol Treat 2023;34(1):2202288.

23. Cheng BT, Silverberg JI. Depression and psychological distress in US adults with atopic dermatitis. Ann Allergy Asthma Immunol 2019;123(2):179–85.

24. Chiesa Fuxench ZC, Block JK, Boguniewicz M, et al. Atopic dermatitis in america study: a cross-sectional study examining the prevalence and disease burden of atopic dermatitis in the US adult population. J Invest Dermatol 2019;139(3):583–90.

25. Sandhu JK, Wu KK, Bui TL, et al. Association between atopic dermatitis and suicidality: a systematic review and meta-analysis. JAMA Dermatol 2019;155(2):178–87.

26. Silverberg JI, Gelfand JM, Margolis DJ, et al. Symptoms and diagnosis of anxiety and depression in atopic dermatitis in U.S. adults. Br J Dermatol 2019;181(3):554–65.

27. Johnson JK, Loiselle AR, Chatrath S, et al. Patient and caregiver perspectives on the relationship between atopic dermatitis symptoms and mental health. Dermatitis 2024. https://doi.org/10.1089/derm.2023.0365.

28. Cheng A, Wan J, Chen SC, et al. Atopic dermatitis and bullying among US adolescents. JAMA Dermatol 2023;159(12):1395–7.

29. Roosta N, Black DS, Peng D, et al. Skin disease and stigma in emerging adulthood: impact on healthy development. J Cutan Med Surg 2010;14(6):285–90.

30. Silverberg JI, Feldman SR, Smith Begolka W, et al. Patient perspectives of atopic dermatitis: comparative analysis of terminology in social media and scientific literature, identified by a systematic literature review. J Eur Acad Dermatol Venereol 2022;36(11): 1980–90.

31. Maleki-Yazdi KA, Heen AF, Zhao IX, et al. Values and preferences of patients and caregivers regarding treatment of atopic dermatitis (eczema): a systematic review. JAMA Dermatol 2023;159(3): 320–30.

32. Chatrath S, LeBovidge J, Jack C, et al. Mental health interventions for atopic dermatitis: knowledge gaps, pilot programmes and future directions. Clin Exp Dermatol 19 2023;49(1):9–17.

33. Lio PA, Wollenberg A, Thyssen JP, et al. Impact of atopic dermatitis lesion location on quality of life in adult patients in a real-world study. J Drugs Dermatol 2020;19(10):943–8.

34. Capozza K, Schwartz A, Lang JE, et al. Impact of childhood atopic dermatitis on life decisions for caregivers and families. J Eur Acad Dermatol Venereol 2022;36(6):e451–4.

35. Cheng BT, Silverberg JI. Association of pediatric atopic dermatitis and psoriasis with school absenteeism and parental work absenteeism: A cross-sectional United States population-based study. J Am Acad Dermatol 2021;85(4):885–92.

36. Misery L, Seneschal J, Corgibet F, et al. Impact of atopic dermatitis on patients and their partners. Acta Derm Venereol 26 2023;103:adv5285.

37. Sibbald C, Drucker AM. Patient burden of atopic dermatitis. Dermatol Clin 2017;35(3):303–16.

38. Drucker AM, Qureshi AA, Amand C, et al. Health care resource utilization and costs among adults with atopic dermatitis in the United States: a claims-based analysis. J Allergy Clin Immunol Pract Jul-2018;6(4):1342–8.

39. Smith Begolka W, Chovatiya R, Thibau IJ, et al. Financial burden of atopic dermatitis out-of-pocket health care expenses in the United States. Dermatitis 2021;32(1S):S62–70.

40. Chovatiya R, Smith Begolka W, Thibau I, et al. Atopic dermatitis polypharmacy and out-of-pocket healthcare expenses. J Drugs Dermatol 2023;22(2): 154–64.

41. Loiselle AR, Thibau IJ, Johnson JK, et al. Financial and treatment access burden associated with atopic dermatitis comorbidities. Ann Allergy Asthma Immunol 2023;(0):0. https://doi.org/10.1016/j.anai.2023. 10.015.

42. Drucker AM, Wang AR, Li WQ, et al. The burden of atopic dermatitis: summary of a report for the National Eczema Association. J Invest Dermatol 2017; 137(1):26–30.

43. Chovatiya R, Begolka WS, Thibau IJ, et al. Impact and Associations of atopic dermatitis out-of-pocket health care expenses in the United States. Dermatitis Nov-01 2022;33(6S):S43–51.

44. Loiselle A, Chovatiya R, Thibau IJ, et al. Evaluating access to prescription medications in the atopic dermatitis patient population. Dermatol Ther 2023 [pending approval].

45. Adams K, Greiner AC, Corrigan JM. *The 1st Annual Crossing the Quality Chasm Summit: A Focus on Communities Institute of Medicine (US) Committee on the Crossing the Quality Chasm: Next Steps Toward a New Health Care.* In: *System.* Washington, DC: National Academies Press (US); 2004.

46. Wilde MH, Garvin S. A concept analysis of self-monitoring. J Adv Nurs 2007;57(3):339–50.

47. Jiang J, Cameron A-F. IT-enabled self-monitoring for chronic disease self-management: an interdisciplinary review. MIS Q 2020;44(1):451–508.

48. McBain H, Shipley M, Newman S. The impact of self-monitoring in chronic illness on healthcare utilisation: a systematic review of reviews. BMC Health Serv Res 2015;15(1):565.

49. Huygens MW, Swinkels IC, de Jong JD, et al. Self-monitoring of health data by patients with a chronic disease: does disease controllability matter? BMC Fam Pract 20 2017;18(1):40.

50. Johnsson N, Strandberg S, Tuvesson H, et al. Delineating and clarifying the concept of self-care monitoring: a concept analysis. Int J Qual Stud Health Well-Being 2023;18(1):2241231.

51. Leshem YA, Chalmers JR, Apfelbacher C, et al. Measuring atopic eczema symptoms in clinical practice: The first consensus statement from the Harmonising Outcome Measures for Eczema in clinical practice initiative. J Am Acad Dermatol 2020; 82(5):1181–6.

52. Williams HC, Schmitt J, Thomas KS, et al. The HOME Core outcome set for clinical trials of atopic dermatitis. J Allergy Clin Immunol 2022;149(6): 1899–911.

53. Thibau I, Begolka WS. 40436 eczema patient and caregiver willingness to engage in a mobile health app for disease management and shared decision making. J Am Acad Dermatol 2023;89(3):AB41.

54. Shah S, Kemp JM, Kvedar JC, et al. A feasibility study of the burden of disease of atopic dermatitis using a smartphone research application. myEczema. Int J Womens Dermatol 2020;6(5):424–8.

55. Gudmundsdottir SL, Ballarini T, Amundadottir ML, et al. Engagement, retention, and acceptability in a digital health program for atopic dermatitis: prospective interventional study. JMIR Form Res 2023; 7:e41227.

56. de Wijs LEM, van Egmond S, Devillers ACA, et al. Needs and preferences of patients regarding atopic dermatitis care in the era of new therapeutic options: a qualitative study. Arch Dermatol Res 2023;315(1): 75–83.

57. van Galen LS, Xu X, Koh MJA, et al. Eczema apps conformance with clinical guidelines: a systematic assessment of functions, tools and content. Br J Dermatol 2020;182(2):444–53.

58. Zvulunov A, Lenevich S, Migacheva N. A mobile health app for facilitating disease management in children with atopic dermatitis: feasibility and impact study. JMIR Dermatol 2023;6(1):e49278.

59. Todorov A, Torah R, Ardern-Jones MR, et al. Electromagnetic sensing techniques for monitoring atopic dermatitis-current practices and possible advancements: a review. Sensors 2023;23(8).

60. Swerlick RA, Zhang C, Patel A, et al. The Skindex-Mini: A streamlined quality of life measurement tool suitable for routine use in clinic. J Am Acad Dermatol 2021;85(2):510–2.

Long-Term Impact of Atopic Dermatitis on Quality of Life

William Fitzmaurice, BS, Nanette B. Silverberg, MD*

KEYWORDS

- Atopic dermatitis • Quality of life • CDLQI • DLQI • SCORAD • PO-SCORAD • IDLQI • POEM

KEY POINTS

- Quality of life in atopic dermatitis is impaired for all age groups, intimate partners, and caretakers.
- Quality of life measurements can be general, creating an easy comparison to other medical diseases, and can be specific to atopic dermatitis by age or region, long or brief, or measure disease longitudinally over time.
- A combination of multiple quality of life scores can yield a multidimensional view into the life alterations experienced by atopic dermatitis patients over the course of their lifetime.

INTRODUCTION

The understanding of the global impact of atopic dermatitis (AD) on the health-related quality of life (HRQoL) of patients was highly advanced by the development of the Hanifin and Rajka criteria for AD in 1980 addressing major and minor criteria that reflect quality of life (QoL).[1] The Dermatology Life Quality Index (DLQI, 1994) and the Children's Dermatology Quality of Life Index (CDLQI, 1995) provide the opportunity to globally and reproducibly assess AD and other skin conditions for their QoL impact.[2–4] Additional concerns were highlighted by scores such as the Patient-Generated Index, which was more focused on sleep and swimming as concerns for AD patients (1997), but is not a commonly used score.[5] The Scoring for Atopic Dermatitis Index's (SCORAD's) entry into the toolbox was one of the first hybrid severity, extent and symptom scores.[6] In 1999, an article addressing psychological concerns in AD highlighted the differences between SCORAD, the DLQI, and the Spielberger State-Trait Anxiety Index identified higher rates of anxiety in AD and lower QoL scores, but noted that psychological

scores and extent of disease scores were required to wholly characterize disease.[6,7] Effects on daily life including work absenteeism[8] and stigmatization ("Questionnaire on Experience with Skin Complaints")[9] highlight daily impairments and the presence of depressive coping style and rumination.[9]

Additional scores enhanced the applicability of tools across individuals and symptoms. The Nottingham Eczema Severity Score (NESS, 1999) added itch and the element of disease course.[10] The CDLQI and DLQI were later enhanced in applicability by validation as the Toddler DLQI, the Infant DLQI, and the Family Dermatitis Index rounding, enhancing applicability to the long-suffering caretaker and to young children.[11,12] The Infants' Dermatitis Quality of Life Index (IDQoL), which addresses ages 0 to 3, demonstrates widespread usage and utility in QoL, topical, as well as systemic interventional studies.[13] A more recent score is the Childhood Atopic Dermatitis Impact Scale (CADIS), which has 5 domains, has good internal reliability, and can demonstrate the QoL benefits of 28 days of treatment and has a brief version, the CADIS Short

Department of Dermatology, Icahn School of Medicine at Mt Sinai, 234 East 85th Street, 5C, New York, NY 10028, USA
* Corresponding author. 5 E 98th Street, 5th Floor, New York, NY 10029.
E-mail address: nanette.silverberg@mountsinai.org

Dermatol Clin 42 (2024) 549–557
https://doi.org/10.1016/j.det.2024.04.005
0733-8635/24/© 2024 Elsevier Inc. All rights reserved.

Form[14]; these scores were developed specifically for children with AD and to provide specific QoL data in younger patients.[15]

General QoL scores help to create cross-measurement with other medical conditions. The 36-Item Short Form Health Survey (SF-36), a general score of QoL was validated in adult AD patients and is negatively impacted by sleeplessness,[16] correlating to impaired physical functioning, bodily pain, general and mental health, social functioning, and vitality.[17] The EQ-5 and Quality of Life questionnaire can be quite helpful when AD overlaps with other allergic symptomatology.[18,19] The Skindex in its longer and shorter versions (the 3-question Skindex mini), and its teen version, was used to address AD with the advantage of spanning usage from teenage to adults and across continents.[20–25]

The sense of well-being is highly personal and cannot only be predicted by cutaneous features. As a result, patient-reported outcomes (PROs) have become vital to studies of patients with AD.[2] DLQI and CDLQI are self-scored, qualifying as PROs. Newer AD PROs include the Patient-Oriented Eczema Measure (POEM) and the Patient-Reported Outcomes Information System (PROMIS).[26,27] The recent Harmonizing Outcome Measures for Eczema initiative agreed upon long-term control domains including QoL and a patient global instrument, with inclusion of itch frequency and intensity.[28] The PROMIS Itch Questionnaire further highlights the utility of addition of itch scores in assessing QoL.[6,29–31] The POEM score has quickly become a favorite in trials, with good sensitivity in QoL changes over as sensitive as 28 days into treatment.[6,30] Focused inventories of AD disease control are newer long-term measures of QoL. These include Atopic Dermatitis Control Tool (ADCT) which looks at 6 AD symptoms over a 1 week time period: days with intense episodes of itching, intensity of bother, problem with sleep, impact on daily activities, and impact on mood or emotions.[7,32]

The burden of AD on QoL includes the association with depressive and anxiety symptoms. A Chinese study using the Depressive, Anxiety, Stress Scales-42, Beck Depression Inventory-13, NESS, and the CDLQI showed AD patients reported depressive (21%), anxiety (33%), and stress (23%) symptoms commonly.[33]

QoL is best addressed for its multifunctional effects on patients by using both the specific skin and general health scores.[34] The choice of tool depends on the age of the patient and the intention of derived data. If one needs a score to compare to a general health condition, the 12-item Short-Form survey or SF-36 is standardized across all diseases. For comparison to other skin diseases, the skin-specific QoL scores DLQI/CDLQI, POEM, or the PROMIS(R) score is meaningful. For addressing AD-specific issues, more specific scores may be needed. Current trends are leaning toward shorter, easier-to-perform scores such as a 3-question version of the ADCT, Skindex, and the SCORAD and the 2-question Patient Health Questionnaire-2.[35,36] The addition of a depression and anxiety score may add to understanding the patient's response to the disease.[35] The following sections will briefly address both age-specific concerns and age-specific data for infants, children, adolescents, and adults, as well as special concerns including genetics, family, and caregivers, and the specific burden of AD therapy.

INFANTS

Infants are a population greatly affected by AD in both prevalence as well as severity. In 2270 children with AD, it was found that 71.3% of them have at least some form of atopy alongside their AD.[37] Children with asthma have a lower QoL score than those without asthma, and visit the emergency department almost twice as frequently. Their caretakers also have significantly lower QoL.[38] The dependency that infants have on family members during their development leads to many family members being directly affected by an infant's disease course and severity. Both the Infant DLQI (IDLQI) and Family DLQI (fDLIQ) are commonly used in the case of infants to assess the burden that AD places on the individual as well as the family. A positive correlation was found between both SCORAD severity with CDLQI in children and fDLIQ scores in mothers.[39] High severity is correlated with more time spent on childcare as well as more work days missed, while improved disease severity correlates with improved QoL.[40–42]

Infants as young as 6 months of age already have detrimental impact on their QoL over age-matched peers.[43] The IDQoL correlates with parental-determined severity, highlighting the benefit of scores in clinical practice in understanding the level of the problem.[44] The Infant Toddler QoL Index was recently validated with more cross-cultural validation initially.[45] However, IDQoL was used in many cultural settings and based on almost 2 decades of usage, it appears very utilitarian for younger children with AD.

PEDIATRIC

Children with AD are statistically more likely to have impaired QoL than controls. Burdens include discomfort; itchiness or soreness; sleep disturbance which affects intellectual functioning, mood, and family psychosocial function; lifestyle alterations in children such as limitations in clothing, sleepovers, swimming, pets, and sports participation; and the amount of time spent on care. Impairments of QoL are considered equal to asthma and diabetes mellitus in children.[46,47] While clothing choices and school function are addressed by CDLQI, in fact other QoL instruments (eg, SF-36) are needed for comparison to other illnesses, and different instruments for family function. To really understand the childhood burden of AD, both quantitative and qualitative QoL instrumentation is needed.[48]

Children cannot be isolated from their families. Families caring for children with AD literally lose sleep, have reduced relationships and psychosocial functioning, and can suffer from work absenteeism, the burden of special diets and changes in household skin care regimens, and the time lost with siblings due to the extreme time-consuming nature of AD. Caring for children affected by AD can be an extremely time-consuming.[49,50] In children ages 5 to 17, an estimate of 2 out of 3 children with AD have sleep disturbance, with higher odds for moderate to severe disease (2.03x).[51]

While QoL is typically assessed using cross-sectional tools, cumulative life course impairment addresses QoL over time. Single-point QoL is important to highlight needs, 2 points or more over time is needed to address interventions, but clearance and long-term health, including early control of physical and psychological comorbidities, the dimension of time, is really the long-term goal of treating children with AD who suffer from birth through adolescence.[52–55]

Longitudinal studies in childhood are limited. A recent study addressed 1-year outcomes in 98 children with AD using SCORAD, CDLQI for greater than 4 years, and IDLQI for 0 to 4 years, with impairment of QoL score due to AD labeled mild (score from 0 to 6), moderate (score from 7 to 12), and severe (score from 13 to 30). Children with less severe AD were more likely to improve than those with moderate-to-severe disease. In this cohort, lower SCORAD was associated with better QoL.[40] In hospitalized children, the burden of disease is more severe and QoL is worse for those children with earlier-onset disease, highlighting the cumulative burden of AD. Infantile-onset cases have more severe allergic diseases including asthma, food allergies, and allergic rhinitis.[56] Over a 3-year study using CDLQI in 133 children (5–16 years), itch (50%), sleep disturbance (47%), treatment (38%), swimming/sports

(29%), and bullying/teasing (<10%) were noted to affect QoL, with the first 2 being worse for children ≤10 years. Girls had a 2.86 times increased issues with clothing and shoes over boys.[57] Interventional studies in children identify that clinical therapy can improve QoL more than placebo.[58]

TEENS

Teens' data are similar to pediatric, even down to family effects.[59] However, there are unique aspects to adolescent health. Adolescents do not always seek care. The BAMSE (Children, Allergy, Environmental, Stockholm, Epidemiology) population-based cohort showed that persistent AD at ages 12, 16, and 24 years was associated with worse EuroQol visual analogue scale and limited health care contact.[60] Additionally, activity such as sports or swimming and clothing impairment remain a concern for adolescents. Finally, the course of life for atopic teens is negatively impacted by AD including the development of self-image, relationships, and fears of intimacy, including the sexual debut.[61]

ADULTS

Adult AD impacts everyday life.[62,63] Half of AD adults feel like they are stigmatized (22), and upwards of 30% feel that they experience work discrimination.[64] One hundred twenty-five adults recruited by a support group responded to DLQI, the Stigmatization and Eczema Questionnaire, the Hospital Anxiety and Depression Scale, the Fear of Negative Evaluation Scale, and the Rosenberg Self-Esteem Scale, highlighting that stigma was associated with psychological problems and poorer QoL. Nearly half had a mood disorder. Stigma and depression accounted for 44.5% of the variance in QoL in this cohort.[65] Respondents with moderate-to-severe AD (N = 1017) reported sleep difficulties (56.6%), depression (70.7%), and anxiety (60.9%)[66] Like teenagers, adults with AD report lifestyle limitations (51.3%), avoidance of social interaction (39.1%), and impacts on activities (43.3%). Itch, dryness, and inflamed skin are the 3 most burdensome AD symptoms.[27]

One additional explanation is genetic burden. In adults carrying an FLG mutation (16.9% of screened) with AD or hand eczema; FLG mutations (R501X, 2282del4, and R2447X) were significantly associated with AD, fissuring of the hands and feet, and actinic keratoses. Studies show mixed effects on QoL with FLG mutation in adults.[67,68] Another explanation is stressors. Patients reported more problems during the pandemic ($P<.05$) regarding pain/discomfort and social relationships, with notable worsening on EuroQoL-5 Dimension-5 level utility, Skindex-16, DLQI, and DLQI-Relevant.[69]

The most commonly used outcome measures in adults are SCORAD, POEM, DLQI, and Numerical Rating Scale (NRS).[70] In clinical practice, adult AD patients can be assessed by Patient-Oriented-SCORAD (PO-SCORAD), PO-SCORAD objective and subjective subscores, NRS-itch, and POEM.[71] In a trial of patients 12 to 75 years of age with moderate to severe AD (AD Up [A Study to Evaluate Upadacitinib in Combination With Topical Corticosteroids in Adolescent and Adult Participants With Moderate to Severe Atopic Dermatitis]), the Worst Pruritus NRS and the Atopic Dermatitis Symptom and Impact scales were validated.[71] The interested reader is referred to the work by Silverberg, and colleagues, 2018, for parameters of severity strata for POEM, DLQI and PO-SCORAD.[27] In 955 patients with AD (age 18–97 years) after 6, 12, 18, and 24 months, the PROMIS Pediatric Global Health score worsened for incremental increases in all QoL (POEM, NRS) and severity indicators (Eczema Area and Severity Index, SCORAD). It was noted in the study that despite longitudinal trends, many patients have fluctuations that can negatively impact QoL.[72–74]

SEXUAL ACTIVITY

Sexual activity can be impacted negatively in the setting of active AD. Differences by race/ethnicity and sex are poorly characterized in the literature.[75] The sexual life of individuals suffering with AD can be greatly impaired as well with a study finding around 39% and 26% prevalence of decreased sexual desire in partners of patients and patients, respectively. A third of partners also believed that AD was contagious.[76] This leads to less sexual desire and further perpetuates the stigmas surrounding AD for those individuals.[77]

SCHOOL PERFORMANCE

AD may interfere with intellectual functioning in school. Children with AD have lower intellectual quotients than those unaffected with AD in a school and cognitive performance study.[78] Among 3132 children with AD, 1544 (67.7%) missed ≥1 day, and 120 (3.9%) and 5 (3.6%) missed ≥15 days (chronically absent) per year due to illness.[78]

WORK PERFORMANCE

The 2020 Adelphi AD Disease Specific Programme completed a survey demonstrating the presence of itch and skin pain is associated with worse POEM scores, daytime sleepiness, worse symptoms, and 14.5% more overall work impairment.[79,80] All AD patients are at risk for reduced work productivity and absenteeism at work. Of 401 individuals who were surveyed, 4.4% were late in, left early, or did not show up 1 or more days per week; 29.5% said a few days every 2 weeks, and 66.1% said a few days per year. Work impairment was around 24.0 days per worker per year.[81] A study of patients in Taiwan demonstrated one-third reported missing work (absenteeism) in the preceding week due to AD, 88.5% of the remaining two-thirds reported impaired work effectiveness (presenteeism), and 92.5% of all participants reported impaired daily activities. Work impairment was greater for moderate to severe than mild AD.[79] A study from 112 patients in Denmark identified that the mean loss of working days due to AD was 5.8 days/6 months, which was 148% of the national average and 38% of the respondents had abstained from a specific education or a job due to AD. As of the year 2006, the investigators indicated that in the years since 1970, "the average number of pension due to AD awarded in Denmark has grown from 4.2 per year for 1970-1976 to 18.0 per year for 1999-2002."[80] The population-based National Health and Wellness Survey (Europe 2016, USA 2015 and 2016) looked at AD in 1098 respondents and demonstrated that work productivity dropped with increasing PO-SCORAD with 2.4, 9.6, and 19.0 hours per week of potential work loss productivity in mild, moderate, and severe AD, respectively.[81] AD causes 3 times more absenteeism.[82] There is reported two-thirds improvement in work-productivity with dupilumab therapy.[83]

THE BURDEN OF THERAPY

The following is a list (by no means comprehensive) of burdens associated with AD therapy: (1) real adverse events, for example, stinging (target-controlled infusion), conjunctivitis (IL4/IL13 inhibitors), renal concerns (cyclosporine); (2) concerns that may become a psychiatric condition, for example, the fear of unnatural agents, and steroid phobia; (3) difficulty discerning reliable resources (eg, reliance on social media for information); (4) time spent applying therapies including emollients; (5) financial burden; and (6) burden of office visits (eg, repeated visits for narrowband ultraviolet B).

Addressing family burden is an important tactic in addressing QoL.[51,84] The fear of steroids, that is, steroid phobia, is found in almost a third of patients, more in women, and can be measured using the Topical Corticosteroid Phobia and the Osnabruck scales.[85–89] Steroid phobia in parents of children with AD can be linked to nonmedical sources of information, including social media, friends, and family.[85,86] Health care providers may participate in steroid phobia and education may not always help.[90,91] Actual side effects and time spent in care can reduce the general sense of well-being of the family, and can trigger early discontinuation and nonadherence.[85,92–95] A 53-item anonymous online survey for adult patients and caregivers of children with AD showed HRQoL for adult patients with AD (driven by 2 domains: pain/discomfort and anxiety/depression) were worse than those reported for asthma and type 2 diabetes in previous studies (0.72; 95% confidence interval, 0.65–0.78). Patients and caregivers reported substantial financial impacts even in countries with government-funded health care systems, though the greatest impact was in the United States. The burden of AD, evaluated as HRQoL detriments, financial impacts, and uncontrolled symptoms, is significant and highest for patients with more severe AD.[51]

FAMILY MEMBERS

AD has the opportunity to greatly affect the family that is caring for an individual with AD. A study of 171 parents of children with AD found that severity of AD was significantly correlated with family QOL.[52] There were some significant predictors of poorer family QOL with those being PO-SCORAD, Patient-Oriented Sleeplessness, and Perceived Stress Scale.[96] AD increases stress and impairs QOL in mothers and caregivers. Moms of children with AD are more depressive, anxious, and characterized their children as positive less frequently. Family burden is greater with AD.[39,97–99] The presence of AD can greatly affect family QOL with an increased severity having a larger effect on QOL and caretaker burden as well as increasing the presence of anxiety and depressive feelings. Lifestyle, emotional consequences, and relationships are impacted by AD.[100] While parents are impacted by children with AD,[101] partners can experience negative QoL including reduced sexual desire.[102]

SUMMARY

There is a plethora of information and tools that can be used to highlight the QoL impairments of patients with AD throughout their lifetime. Being mindful of the stage of life, growth and development, and the potential impairments by age can help the clinician and researcher focus on appropriate tools and analyses. While scores are all meaningful, improving longitudinal life course is the ultimate goal of all analyses.

CLINICS CARE POINTS

- Quality of life expresses a fluid state of capacity to participate meaningfully in daily activities of life.
- Quality of life in atopic dermatitis can be examined and scored using scoring instruments that have been developed for clinicl and research purposes.
- Quality of life can be measured in all age groups, as well as in a singular moment, over the short-term, and even over the long-term. Combning scoring tools can address can address the experience of atopic dermatitis.

REFERENCES

1. Hanifin JM, Rajka G. Diagnostic features of atopic dermatitis. Acta Derm Venereol 1980;92(suppl): 44–7.
2. Finlay AY, Basra MKA, Piguet V, et al. Dermatology life quality index (DLQI): a paradigm shift to patient-centered outcomes. J Invest Dermatol 2012;132(10):2464–5.
3. Lewis-Jones MS, Finlay AY. The children's dermatology life quality index (CDLQI): initial validation and practical use. Br J Dermatol 1995;132(6): 942–9.
4. Leshem YA, Chalmers JR, Apfelbacher C, et al. Measuring atopic eczema control and itch intensity in clinical practice: a consensus statement from the harmonising outcome measures for eczema in clinical practice (HOME-CP) initiative. JAMA Dermatol 2022;158(12):1429–35.
5. Herd RM, Tidman MJ, Ruta DA, et al. Measurement of quality of life in atopic dermatitis: correlation and validation of two different methods. Br J Dermatol 1997;136(4):502–7. PMID: 9155948.
6. Ridd MJ, Gaunt DM, Guy RH, et al. Comparison of patient (POEM), observer (EASI, SASSAD, TIS) and corneometry measures of emollient effectiveness in children with eczema: findings from the COMET feasibility trial. Br J Dermatol 2018; 179(2):362–70.
7. Bender BG, Ballard R, Canono B, et al. Disease severity, scratching, and sleep quality in patients with atopic dermatitis. J Am Acad Dermatol 2008; 58(3):415–20.
8. Yano C, Saeki H, Ishiji T, et al. Impact of disease severity on work productivity and activity impairment in Japanese patients with atopic dermatitis. J Dermatol 2013;40(9):736–9. Epub 2013 Jul 9. PMID: 23834561.

9. Schmid-Ott G, Kuensebeck HW, Jaeger B, et al. Validity study for the stigmatization experience in atopic dermatitis and psoriatic patients. Acta Derm Venereol 1999;79(6):443–7. PMID: 10598757.

10. Emerson RM, Charman CR, Williams HC. The Nottingham Eczema Severity Score:preliminary refinement of the Rajka and Langeland grading. Br J Dermatol 2000;142(2):288–97. PMID: 10730763.

11. Chernyshov PV, Kaliuzhna LD, Reznikova AA, et al. Comparison of the impairment of family quality of life assessed by disease-specific and dermatology-specific instruments in children with atopic dermatitis. J Eur Acad Dermatol Venereol 2015;29(6):1221–4.

12. Lewis-Jones MS, Finlay AY, Dykes PJ. The infants' dermatitis quality of life index. Br J Dermatol 2001;144(1):104–10. PMID: 11167690.

13. Basra MK, Gada V, Ungaro S, et al. Infants' dermatitis quality of life index: a decade of experience of validation and clinical application. Br J Dermatol 2013;169(4):760–8.

14. Chamlin SL, Lai JS, Cella D, et al. Childhood atopic dermatitis impact scale: reliability, discriminative and concurrent validity, and responsiveness. Arch Dermatol 2007;143(6):768–72.

15. Gabes M, Chamlin SL, Lai JS, et al. Development of a validated short-form of the childhood atopic dermatitis impact scale, the CADIS-SF15. J Eur Acad Dermatol Venereol 2020;34(8):1773–8.

16. Lundberg L, Johannesson M, Silverdahl M, et al. Health-related quality of life in patients with psoriasis and atopic dermatitis measured with SF-36, DLQI and a subjective measure of disease activity. Acta Derm Venereol 2000; 80(6):430–4.

17. Holm EA, Wulf HC, Stegmann H, et al. Life quality assessment among patients with atopic eczema. Br J Dermatol 2006;154(4):719–25.

18. Lee SH, Lee SH, Lee SY, et al. Psychological health status and health-related quality of life in adults with atopic dermatitis: a Nationwide cross-sectional study in South Korea. Acta Derm Venereol 2018;98(1):89–97.

19. Finlay AY. Quality of life assessments in dermatology. Semin Cutan Med Surg 1998;17(4):291–6.

20. Terreehorst I, Duivenvoorden HJ, Tempels-Pavlica Z, et al. The unfavorable effects of concomitant asthma and sleeplessness due to the atopic eczema/dermatitis syndrome (AEDS) on quality of life in subjects allergic to house-dust mites. Allergy 2002;57(10):919–25.

21. Anderson RT, Rajagopalan R. Effects of allergic dermatosis on health-related quality of life. Curr Allergy Asthma Rep 2001;1(4):309–15.

22. Carvalho D, Aguiar P, Ferrinho P. Skindex-29 cutoffs in an atopic dermatitis sample. Int J Dermatol 2021;60(2):e45–7.

23. Dizon MP, Topham C, Haynes D, et al. Validity of the Skindex Mini in Patients With Atopic Dermatitis. Dermatitis 2022;33(6S):S131–3.

24. Higaki Y, Kawamoto K, Kamo T, et al. Measurement of the impact of atopic dermatitis on patients' quality of life: a cross-sectional and longitudinal questionnaire study using the Japanese version of Skindex-16. J Dermatol 2004;31(12):977–82.

25. Sheth AP, Blumstein AJ, Rangel SM, et al. Three-question Skindex-Mini measures quality of life in children with atopic dermatitis. J Am Acad Dermatol 2023;88(2):493–5.

26. Silverberg JI, Lei D, Yousaf M, et al. Comparison of patient-oriented eczema measure and patient-oriented scoring atopic dermatitis vs eczema area and severity index and other measures of atopic dermatitis: a validation study. Ann Allergy Asthma Immunol 2020;125(1):78–83.

27. Silverberg JI, Gelfand JM, Margolis DJ, et al. Severity strata for POEM, PO-SCORAD, and DLQI in US adults with atopic dermatitis. Ann Allergy Asthma Immunol 2018;121(4):464–8.e3.

28. Chalmers JR, Thomas KS, Apfelbacher C, et al. Report from the fifth international consensus meeting to harmonize core outcome measures for atopic eczema/dermatitis clinical trials (HOME initiative). Br J Dermatol 2018;178(5):e332–41.

29. Silverberg JI, Lai JS, Kantor RW, et al. Development, validation, and interpretation of the PROMIS itch questionnaire: a patient-reported outcome measure for the quality of life impact of itch. J Invest Dermatol 2020;140(5):986–94.e6.

30. Silverberg JI, Chiesa Fuxench ZC, Gelfand JM, et al. Content and construct validity, predictors, and distribution of self-reported atopic dermatitis severity in US adults. Ann Allergy Asthma Immunol 2018;121(6):729–34.e4.

31. Leshem YA, Chalmers JR, Apfelbacher C, et al. Harmonising Outcome Measures for Eczema (HOME) initiative. measuring atopic eczema control and itch intensity in clinical practice: a consensus statement from the harmonising outcome measures for eczema in clinical practice (HOME-CP) Initiative. JAMA Dermatol 2022; 158(12):1429–35.

32. Simpson E, Eckert L, Gadkari A, et al. Validation of the Atopic Dermatitis Control Tool (ADCT©) using a longitudinal survey of biologic-treated patients with atopic dermatitis. BMC Dermatol 2019;19(1):15. PMID: 31690295; PMCID: PMC6833284.

33. Hon KL, Pong NH, Poon TC, et al. Quality of life and psychosocial issues are important outcome measures in eczema treatment. J Dermatol Treat 2015;26(1):83–9.

34. Maksimović N, Janković S, Marinković J, et al. Health-related quality of life in patients with atopic dermatitis. J Dermatol 2012;39(1):42–7.

35. Silverberg JI, Lee B, Lei D, et al. Measurement properties of patient health questionnaire 9 and patient health questionnaire 2 in adult patients with atopic dermatitis. Dermatitis : Contact, Atopic, Occupational, Drug 2021;32(4):225–31. PMID: 33273219.

36. van Oosterhout M, Janmohamed SR, Spierings M, et al. Correlation between Objective SCORAD and Three-Item Severity Score used by physicians and Objective PO-SCORAD used by parents/patients in children with atopic dermatitis. Dermatology 2015;230(2):105–12.

37. Kapoor R, Menon C, Hoffstad O, et al. The prevalence of atopic triad in children with physician-confirmed atopic dermatitis. J Am Acad Dermatol 2008;58(1):68–73.

38. Agrawal S, Iqbal S, Patel SJ, et al. Quality of life in at-risk school-aged children with asthma. J Asthma 2021;58(12):1680–8.

39. Kilic N, Kilic M. Investigation of quality of life of patients with atopic dermatitis and quality of life, psychiatric symptomatology, and caregiver burden of their mothers. Children 2023;10(9):1487.

40. Gazibara T, Reljic V, Jankovic S, et al. Quality of life in children with atopic dermatitis: A one-year prospective cohort study. Indian J Dermatol Venereol Leprol 2021;88(1):65–9.

41. Barbarot S, Silverberg JI, Gadkari A, et al. The family impact of atopic dermatitis in the pediatric population: results from an international cross-sectional study. J Pediatr 2022;246:220–6.e5.

42. Salava A, Perälä M, Juppo M, et al. Effective treatment of atopic dermatitis in small children significantly improves the quality of life of patients and their families. Eur J Dermatol 2021;31(6):791–7.

43. Alanne S, Nermes M, Söderlund R, et al. Quality of life in infants with atopic dermatitis and healthy infants: a follow-up from birth to 24 months. Acta Paediatr 2011;100(8):e65–70.

44. van Valburg RW, Willemsen MG, Dirven-Meijer PC, et al. Quality of life measurement and its relationship to disease severity in children with atopic dermatitis in general practice. Acta Derm Venereol 2011;91(2):147–51.

45. Chernyshov PV, Sampogna F, Pustišek N, et al. Validation of the dermatology-specific proxy instrument the Infants and Toddlers Dermatology Quality of Life. J Eur Acad Dermatol Venereol 2019;33(7):1405–11.

46. Lewis-Jones S. Quality of life and childhood atopic dermatitis: the misery of living with childhood eczema. Int J Clin Pract 2006;60(8):984–92.

47. Beattie PE, Lewis-Jones MS. A comparative study of impairment of quality of life in children with skin disease and children with other chronic childhood diseases. Br J Dermatol 2006;155(1):145–51.

48. Chamlin SL, Chren MM. Quality-of-life outcomes and measurement in childhood atopic dermatitis. Immunol Allergy Clin 2010;30(3):281–8. Epub 2010 Jul 1. PMID: 20670813; PMCID: PMC3150535.

49. Yang EJ, Beck KM, Sekhon S, et al. The impact of pediatric atopic dermatitis on families: A review. Pediatr Dermatol 2019;36(1):66–71.

50. Capozza Korey, Funk Melanie, Hering Marjolaine, et al. Patients' and Caregivers' Experiences With Atopic Dermatitis–Related Burden, Medical Care, and Treatments in 8 Countries. J Allergy Clin Immunol Pract 2023;11(1):264–73. e1, ISSN 2213-2198.

51. Fishbein AB, Cheng BT, Tilley CC, et al. Sleep disturbance in school-aged children with atopic dermatitis: prevalence and severity in a cross-sectional sample. J Allergy Clin Immunol Pract 2021;9(8):3120–9.e3.

52. Finlay AY. Quality of life in atopic dermatitis. J Am Acad Dermatol 2001;45(1 Suppl):S64–6.

53. von Stülpnagel CC, Augustin M, Düpmann L, et al. Mapping risk factors for cumulative life course impairment in patients with chronic skin diseases - a systematic review. J Eur Acad Dermatol Venereol 2021;35(11):2166–84.

54. Stangier U, Ehlers A, Gieler U. Predicting long-term outcome in group treatment of atopic dermatitis. Psychother Psychosom 2004;73(5):293–301.

55. Ražnatović Đurović M, Janković J, Tomić Spirić V, et al. Does age influence the quality of life in children with atopic dermatitis? PLoS One 2019;14(11):e0224618. PMID: 31725802; PMCID: PMC6855426.

56. Jeon YH, Ahn K, Kim J, et al. Food Allergy and Atopic Dermatitis (FAAD) Study Group in the Korean Academy of Pediatric Allergy and Respiratory Disease. Clinical Characteristics of Atopic Dermatitis in Korean School-Aged Children and Adolescents According to Onset Age and Severity. J Kor Med Sci 2022;37(4):e30. PMID: 35075829; PMCID: PMC8787802.

57. Hon KL, Leung TF, Wong KY, et al. Does age or gender influence quality of life in children with atopic dermatitis? Clin Exp Dermatol 2008;33(6):705–9.

58. McKenna SP, Whalley D, de Prost Y, et al. Treatment of paediatric atopic dermatitis with pimecrolimus (Elidel, SDZ ASM 981): impact on quality of life and health-related quality of life. J Eur Acad Dermatol Venereol 2006;20(3):248–54.

59. Amaral CS, March Mde F, Sant'Anna CC. Quality of life in children and teenagers with atopic dermatitis. An Bras Dermatol 2012;87(5):717–23.

60. Lundin S, Jonsson M, Wahlgren CF, et al. Young adults' perceptions of living with atopic dermatitis in relation to the concept of self-management: a qualitative study. BMJ Open 2021;11(6):e044777.

61. Brenninkmeijer EE, Legierse CM, Sillevis Smitt JH, et al. The course of life of patients with childhood

atopic dermatitis. Pediatr Dermatol 2009;26(1): 14–22.

62. Asher MI, Montefort S, Björkstén B, et al. World-wide time trends in the prevalence of symptoms of asthma, allergic rhinoconjunctivitis, and eczema in childhood: ISAAC Phases One and Three repeat multicountry cross-sectional surveys [published correction appears in Lancet. 2007 Sep 29; 370(9593):1128]. Lancet 2006;368(9537):733–43.

63. Angles MV, Antonietti CA, Torre AC, et al. Prevalence of atopic dermatitis in adults. An Bras Dermatol 2022;97(1):107–9.

64. Stingeni L, Belloni Fortina A, Baiardini I, et al. Atopic dermatitis and patient perspectives: insights of bullying at school and career discrimination at work. J Asthma Allergy 2021;14:919–28. PMID: 34321892; PMCID: PMC8312319.

65. Wittkowski A, Richards HL, Griffiths CE, et al. The impact of psychological and clinical factors on quality of life in individuals with atopic dermatitis. J Psychosom Res 2004;57(2):195–200.

66. Kwatra SG, Gruben D, Fung S, et al. Psychosocial comorbidities and health status among adults with moderate-to-severe atopic dermatitis: A 2017 US National Health and Wellness Survey Analysis. Adv Ther 2021;38(3):1627–37. Epub 2021 Feb 8. PMID: 33555555; PMCID: PMC7932976.

67. Heede NG, Thyssen JP, Thuesen BH, et al. Health-related quality of life in adult dermatitis patients stratified by filaggrin genotype. Contact Dermatitis 2017;76(3):167–77.

68. Holm JG, Agner T, Clausen ML, et al. Quality of life and disease severity in patients with atopic dermatitis. J Eur Acad Dermatol Venereol 2016;30(10): 1760–7.

69. Koszorú K, Hajdu K, Brodszky V, et al. General and skin-specific health-related quality of life in patients with atopic dermatitis before and during the COVID-19 Pandemic. Dermatitis 2022;33(6S): S92–103. Epub 2022 Jun 8. PMID: 35674639; PMCID: PMC9674441.

70. Gooderham MJ, Hong CH, Albrecht L, et al. Approach to the assessment and management of adult patients with atopic dermatitis: a consensus document. J Cutan Med Surg 2018;22(1_suppl): 3S–5S.

71. Silverberg JI, Leshem YA, Calimlim BM, et al. Psychometric evaluation of the Worst Pruritus Numerical Rating Scale (NRS), Atopic Dermatitis Symptom Scale (ADerm-SS), and Atopic Dermatitis Impact Scale (ADerm-IS). Curr Med Res Opin 2023;39(10):1289–96.

72. Schwartzman G, Lei D, Ahmed A, et al. Longitudinal course and phenotypes of health-related quality of life in adults with atopic dermatitis. Clin Exp Dermatol 2022;47(2):359–72.

73. Zachariae R, Zachariae C, Ibsen HH, et al. Psychological symptoms and quality of life of dermatology outpatients and hospitalized dermatology patients. Acta Derm Venereol 2004;84(3):205–12.

74. Paul C, Griffiths CEM, Costanzo A, et al. Factors predicting quality of life impairment in adult patients with atopic dermatitis: results from a patient survey and machine learning analysis. Dermatol Ther 2023;13(4):981–95. Epub 2023 Mar 2. PMID: 36862306; PMCID: PMC10060474.

75. Birdi G, Cooke R, Knibb RC. Impact of atopic dermatitis on quality of life in adults: a systematic review and meta-analysis. Int J Dermatol 2020; 59(4):e75–91.

76. Misery L, Seneschal J, Corgibet F, et al. Impact of Atopic Dermatitis on Patients and their Partners. Acta Derm Venereol 2023;103:adv5285.

77. Torisu-Itakura H, Anderson P, Piercy J, et al. Impact of itch and skin pain on quality of life in adult patients with atopic dermatitis in Japan: results from a real-world, point-in-time, survey of physicians and patients. Curr Med Res Opin 2022;38(8): 1401–10.

78. Vittrup I, Andersen YMF, Skov L, et al. The association between atopic dermatitis, cognitive function and school performance in children and young adults. Br J Dermatol 2023;188(3):341–9.

79. Chan TC, Lin YC, Cho YT, et al. Impact of atopic dermatitis on work and activity impairment in Taiwan. Acta Derm Venereol 2021;101(9): adv00556.

80. Holm EA, Esmann S, Jemec GB. The handicap caused by atopic dermatitis–sick leave and job avoidance. J Eur Acad Dermatol Venereol 2006; 20(3):255–9.

81. Andersen L, Nyeland ME, Nyberg F. Increasing severity of atopic dermatitis is associated with a negative impact on work productivity among adults with atopic dermatitis in France, Germany, the U.K. and the U.S.A. Br J Dermatol 2020;182(4): 1007–16. Epub 2019 Sep 8. PMID: 31260080; PMCID: PMC7187138.

82. Eckert L, Gupta S, Amand C, et al. Impact of atopic dermatitis on health-related quality of life and productivity in adults in the United States: An analysis using the National Health and Wellness Survey. J Am Acad Dermatol 2017;77(2):274–9.e3.

83. Ariëns LFM, Bakker DS, Spekhorst LS, et al. Rapid and sustained effect of dupilumab on work productivity in patients with difficult-to-treat atopic dermatitis: results from the Dutch BioDay Registry. Acta Derm Venereol 2021;101(10): adv00573.

84. Carroll CL, Balkrishnan R, Feldman SR, et al. The burden of atopic dermatitis: impact on the patient, family, and society. Pediatr Dermatol 2005;22(3): 192–9.

85. Fitzmaurice W, Silverberg NB. Systematic review of steroid phobia in atopic dermatitis". Dermatitis 2024. https://doi.org/10.1089/derm.2023.0213.

86. Song SY, Jung SY, Kim E. Steroid phobia among general users of topical steroids: a cross-sectional nationwide survey. J Dermatol Treat 2019;30(3):245–50.

87. Kotarski O, Pečnjak M, Blekić M, et al. The impact of atopic dermatitis and corticophobia on the quality of family life. Acta Dermatovenerol Croat 2023; 31(1):3–10.

88. Yin LJ, Wei TK, Choi E, et al. TOPICOP© scale for steroid phobia - difficulties and suggestions for application in clinical research. J Dermatol Treat 2020;31(6):624–5.

89. Starbek Zorko M, Benko M, Rakuša M, et al. Evaluation of corticophobia in patients with atopic dermatitis and psoriasis using the TOPICOP© score. Acta Dermatovenerol Alpina Pannonica Adriatica 2023;32(4):135–9.

90. Bos B, Antonescu I, Osinga H, et al. Corticosteroid phobia (corticophobia) in parents of young children with atopic dermatitis and their health care providers. Pediatr Dermatol 2019;36(1):100–4.

91. Feldman SR, Huang WW. Steroid phobia isn't reduced by improving patients' knowledge of topical corticosteroids. J Am Acad Dermatol 2020;83(6):e403–4.

92. Nickles MA, Coale AT, Henderson WJA, et al. Steroid phobia on social media platforms. Pediatr Dermatol 2023;40(3):479–82.

93. Rao VU, Apter AJ. Steroid phobia and adherence–problems, solutions, impact on benefit/risk profile. Immunol Allergy Clin 2005;25(3):581–95.

94. Balieva FN, Finlay AY, Kupfer J, et al. The role of therapy in impairing quality of life in dermatological patients: a multinational study. Acta Derm Venereol 2018;98(6):563–9.

95. Jemec GB, Esmann S, Holm EA, et al. Time spent on treatment (TSOT). An independent assessment of disease severity in atopic dermatitis. Acta Dermatovenerol Alpina Pannonica Adriatica 2006; 15(3):119–24.

96. Pustišek N, Vurnek Živković M, Šitum M. Quality of life in families with children with atopic dermatitis. Pediatr Dermatol 2016;33(1):28–32.

97. Kobusiewicz AK, Tarkowski B, Kaszuba A, et al. The relationship between atopic dermatitis and atopic itch in children and the psychosocial functioning of their mothers: A cross-sectional ,study. Front Med 2023;10:1066495.

98. Kobusiewicz AK, Tarkowski B, Kaszuba A, et al. Strategies forcoping with stress in mothers of children with atopic dermatitis - a cross-sectional study. Postepy Dermatol Alergol 2023;40(5):630–7.

99. Pauli-Pott U, Darui A, Beckmann D. Infants with atopic dermatitis: maternal hopelessness, child-rearing attitudes and perceived infant temperament. Psychother Psychosom 1999;68(1):39–45.

100. Snyder AM, Brandenberger AU, Taliercio VL, et al. Quality of life among family of patients with atopic dermatitis and psoriasis. Int J Behav Med 2023; 30(3):409–15.

101. Ražnatović Đurović M, Janković J, Ćirković A, et al. Impact of atopic dermatitis on the quality of life of children and their families. Ital J Dermatol Venerol 2021;156(1):29–35.

102. Misery L, Finlay AY, Martin N, et al. Atopic dermatitis: impact on the quality of life of patients and their partners. Dermatology 2007;215(2):123–9.

VINDICATE-P
A Mnemonic for the Many Comorbidities of Atopic Dermatitis

Nanette B. Silverberg, MD[a],*, Mary F. Lee-Wong, MD, MS, MSc[b],
Jonathan I. Silverberg, MD, PhD, MPH[c]

KEYWORDS

- Atopic dermatitis • Asthma • Food allergies • Allergic rhinoconjunctivitis • Eosinophilic esophagitis

KEY POINTS

- Atopic dermatitis (AD) is a chronic inflammatory skin disease that is associated with many comorbidities that fall under a variety of subtypes.
- Comorbidities may vary with age, but almost every individual with AD will one day develop a comorbidity.
- Comorbidities of AD can be categorized under the mnemonic VINDICATE-P: *v*ascular/cardiovascular, *i*nfectious, *n*eoplastic and *n*eurologic, *d*egenerative, *i*atrogenic, *c*ongenital, *a*topic and *a*utoimmune, *t*raumatic, *e*ndocrine/metabolic, and *p*sychiatric.

INTRODUCTION

The concept of comorbidities was recognized in atopic dermatitis (AD) for many decades. A review article discussing "infantile eczema" published in 1946 wrote "eczematous infants may exchange their skin condition for asthma or hay fever, as they get older"[1] which has been coined the "allergic march."[2] Many of these eczematous infants with chronic AD of childhood, will later in adolescence and adult life have positive skin tests to proteins.[2] While the concept of comorbidities is certainly not new, our knowledge of specific comorbidities, the epidemiology, and burden certainly expanded over time. An early list of recognized comorbidities was considered minor AD criteria by Hanifin and Rajka in 1979.[3] To create a more organized scaffold of the myriad comorbidities, we developed a new mnemonic for this article—"VINDICATE-P":

*v*ascular/cardiovascular, *i*nfectious, *n*eoplastic and *n*eurologic, *d*egenerative, *i*atrogenic, congenital, *a*topic and *a*utoimmune, *t*raumatic, endocrine/metabolic, and *p*sychiatric comorbidities (**Box 1**).

There are age-related differences in the epidemiology of comorbidities associated with AD. Overall, pediatric patients were found to more commonly have impetigo, folliculitis, seborrheic dermatitis, chronic and acute urticaria, lichen nitidus and lichn striatus, and bronchial asthma.[4] In particular, studies examining the frequency of minor Hanifin-Rajka criteria demonstrated infections to be more common in children with AD ages 2 to 12 versus less than 2 year old. Children and adolescents seem more prone to neuropsychiatric comorbidities, for example, migraines, and autoimmune conditions, for example, vitiligo, which is notably associated with AD in children under

[a] Department of Dermatology, Icahn School of Medicine at Mount Sinai, 5 East 98th Street, 5th Floor, New York, NY 10028, USA; [b] Division of Adult Allergy and Immunology, Maimonides Medical Center, 4813 9th Avenue, 5th Floor, Brooklyn, NY 11219, USA; [c] Department of Dermatology, George Washington University School of Medicine and Health Sciences, 2150 Pennsylvania Avenue Northwest, Suite 2B-430, Washington, DC 20037, USA
* Corresponding author.
E-mail address: Nanette.silverberg@mountsinai.org

Dermatol Clin 42 (2024) 559–567
https://doi.org/10.1016/j.det.2024.04.006
0733-8635/24/© 2024 Elsevier Inc. All rights reserved.

derm.theclinics.com

Box 1
The VINDICATE-P mnemonic

Vascular/cardiovascular[6-8] (Risk begins in adulthood[9])

- Coronary artery disease
- Ischemic stroke
- Heart attack
- Congestive heart failure
- Hypertension

Infectious[10-18] (Risk is lifetime[18])

  Bacterial

- Impetigo
- Abscesses
- Erysipelas/cellulitis
- Sore throat
- Strep throat
- Pneumonia
- Urinary tract infections
- Recurrent ear infections
- Sinus infections
- Bacterial conjunctivitis
- Septicemia

  Fungal

- IgE to Malassezia

  Viral

- Warts
- Molluscum
- Varicella
- Herpes zoster
- Extra-genital herpes
- Condyloma
- Eczema herpeticum
- Eczema coxsackium
- Eczema vaccinatum
- Head or chest colds
- Influenza

Neoplastic[19,20] (Risk occurs lifetime[19])

- Non-CTCL lymphoma
- Skin cancer

Neurologic[21,22] (Risk occurs lifetime[21,22])

- Epilepsy
- Headaches/migraines

Degenerative[18,23-26] (Risk identified in middle to late adulthood[27])

  Osteoporosis

  Enthesopathy

  Intravertebral disk disorders

Iatrogenic[29]

  Osteoporosis

  Immunosuppression

  Cancer from phototherapy

  Ocular surface disease

  Drug-induced cataracts

Congenital[2,30-32] (Risk begins at birth)

  Ocular

- Keratoconus
- Anterior subcapsular cataracts

  Cutaneous

- Ichthyosis vulgaris
- Xerosis
- Keratosis pilaris

Atopic and autoimmune[5,35-41] (Risk of atopic comorbidities continuous throughout lifespan)

- Asthma
- Food allergies
- Allergic rhinoconjunctivitis
- EOE
- Allergic contact dermatitis
- Chronic urticaria[42]
- Granuloma annulare[52]
- Rosacea[19]
- Vitiligo[47-49]
- Alopecia areata[19]

Traumatic[55,56]

  Falls

Endocrine/metabolic[5,58-60] (Risk of comorbidity starts in early childhood and progresses through life)

  Diabetes type 2

  Metabolic Syndrome

  Non-alcoholic fatty liver

Psychiatric[61-63] (Risk of comorbidity continuous through life)

  Depression

  Anxiety

  Sleep disorder

  Sleep apnea

  ADHD

  Dementia

Abbreviations: ADHD, attention deficit hyperactivity disorder; CTCL, cutaneous T-cell lymphoma; EOE, eosinophilic esophagitis.

12 years. In adulthood, AD was found to be associated with endocrine/metabolic disorders, for example, metabolic syndrome and type 2 diabetes; slight increase in risk for some neoplastic disorders, including non-cutaneous T-cell lymphomas (non-CTCLs) and skin cancers; and vascular/cardiovascular conditions, for example, hypertension, myocardial infarction, coronary artery disease (CAD), and stroke, particularly in moderate to severe AD. Geriatric patients with more severe AD may particularly have increased risk of dementia and osteoporosis. Psychiatric conditions, for example, depression and anxiety, are overrepresented in adults, while attention-deficit disorder is higher in teens. Traumatic and iatrogenic events can occur at any age. The wide array of comorbidities illustrates that AD can pervasively impact many aspects of health beyond the skin. The recent American Academy of Dermatology (AAD) guidelines on AD comorbidities in adults made clear statements of association of AD in adults with allergic conditions, immune-mediated conditions, mental health and substance abuse, cardiovascular disease, metabolic disorders, bone health, and skin infections.[5] We expect that this list will continue to grow over time and be a starting point, rather than a compendium.

VASCULAR AND CARDIOVASCULAR COMORBIDITIES

Although it is clearly a concern of adulthood, ultimately cardiovascular disease can shorten life expectancy and was the leading cause of death in the United States for 100 years.[6] Analysis of data from the United States population-based 2005 to 2006 National Health and Nutrition Examination Survey, 2010 and 2012 National Health Interview Surveys found associations of flexural eczema with increased odd of CAD, heart attack, congestive heart failure, peripheral vascular disease, and stroke in at least 1 study.[7] A Taiwanese population-based study found a 33% increase in the odds of ischemic stroke in AD patients overall, and 71% increased odds in patients with severe AD.[8] In the All of Us Research Program, hypertension (odds ratio [OR] = 1.56) and hyperlipidemia (OR = 2.29) were associated with AD in multivariate analysis, supporting an association with AD.[9] A systematic review of cardiovascular risk in children with AD found no significant association of AD with diabetes, hypertension, or ischemic heart disease.[10] Thus, it appears that increased screening for cardiovascular risk may not be warranted in children and may have a higher yield in late adolescence and adulthood.

INFECTIONS

Cutaneous and extracutaneous infections are quite common in young children with or without AD. Malassezia sensitization with the production of immunoglobulin E (IgE)[11] and Molluscum contagiosum infections[12] were linked to AD onset in infancy and early childhood, respectively. Wild-type varicella zoster virus (VZV) may protect against developing AD[13,14] but is still associated with severe exacerbation of preexisting AD when generalized as a varicelliform eruption.[15] Cutaneous viral (warts, molluscum, herpesvirus) and bacterial (impetigo) infections, were linked to AD.[3] Analysis of the 2007 National Health Interview Survey showed higher odds of warts in US children with AD.[16] AD was also associated with extracutaneous infections including strep throat, sore throat, head or chest cold, influenza/pneumonia, sinus infections, recurrent ear infections, chickenpox, and urinary tract infections.[16] Recently, eczema coxsackium, a widespread severe spread of coxsackie lesions across the skin in children with AD, was more frequently observed.[17] IgE production to Malassezia increases with age and peaks at ages 20 to 30 years.[18] A large study of Finnish adults identified many comorbidities including abscesses, erysipelas/cellulitis, impetigo, herpes zoster, extragenital herpes, bacterial conjunctivitis, condylomas, and septicemia.[19] Similar pediatric and adult AD data in the US show higher odds of carbuncles/furuncles, impetigo, cellulitis, erysipelas, Staphylococcus aureus infection (methicillin-resistant Staphylococcus aureus and methicillin-susceptible Staphylococcus aureus), molluscum, cutaneous warts, herpes simplex virus (HSV) and VZV, eczema herpeticum, dermatophytosis, and candidiasis of the skin/nails and vulva/urogenitals.[20] Specific to adults are the increased risk of genital HSV infections and genital warts.[20] Together, risk of cutaneous and extracutaneous infections is increased in persons with AD at all ages.

NEOPLASTIC

Linkage of neoplastic disease to AD is important. However, without understanding the baseline risk of neoplasms, it is difficult to appreciate the additional risk conveyed by various treatment modalities. Analysis of The Health Improvement Network from 1994 to 2015 found that children with severe AD had increased risk of non-CTCL lymphoma, and those with mild AD had increased non-melanoma skin cancer (NMSC) risk; adults had 2-fold increased odds of non-CTCL lymphoma and mild increases in NMSC.[21] A systematic review and meta-analysis also concluded that AD is associated with lymphoma due to high-potency topical corticosteroid usage.[21] AD was not found to be consistently associated with solid tumors. One study suggested there may even be a lower odd of solid tumors in patients with AD.[21]

NEUROLOGIC

The US population-based National Survey of Children's Health 2007 to 2008 found that children with an atopic disease, including asthma, AD, hay fever, and food allergies had higher odds of epilepsy; severe AD was associated with an even higher risk.[22] Migraines were linked to AD in children and adults, with potential mechanism of occurrence being interleukin-4 (IL-4) release.[19,23–26]

DEGENERATIVE COMORBIDITIES

Osteoporosis and degenerative disk disease were linked to AD in adults.[19] It is unclear whether this is a cumulative risk caused by long-term usage of topical high-potency and systemic corticosteroids.[27] However, recent data on short-term 2-week to 6-week usage of the class 2 topical corticosteroid betamethasone did not affect bone mineral turnover.[28] Osteoporosis and bone mineral alterations do not appear to be more common in young adults with AD.[29] Data in children are reassuring that usage of topical corticosteroids does not increase risk of fractures in AD patients.[30] However, osteoporosis is a well-established adverse event of systemic corticosteroids. Due to the terrible adverse event profile, systemic corticosteroids are not recommended for AD treatment. The role of vitamin D deficiency and supplementation is also being explored. Vitamin D may have immunomodulatory impact on inflammatory pathways activated by allergic responses. Some studies have suggested that vitamin D supplementation may help prevent allergic diseases.[31,32]

IATROGENIC COMORBIDITIES

One of the consequences of treating AD patients is that therapies can induce comorbidities, the so-called iatrogenic comorbidities. A list of all these adverse-effects is beyond the scope of this review, but merits consideration in the choice of therapeutic agents, and treatment decision-making to reduce risk of adverse events over time. Current guidelines for systemic medications and phototherapy in AD highlight some of the associated risks.[33]

CONGENITAL (AND EARLY-ONSET) COMORBIDITIES

The comorbid conditions of AD seen in early childhood include some of the minor features including ichthyosis vulgaris, keratosis pilaris, keratoconus, and subcapsular cataracts.

An Indian cohort of children highlighted several congenital comorbidities of childhood AD, including xerosis, Dennie-Morgan fold, palmar hyper-linearity, ichthyosis vulgaris, keratosis pilaris, and orbital darkening.[34] These comorbidities of early childhood may be destined to occur from birth and promoted by environmental factors. Filaggrin null mutations are inherited in an autosomal semidominant manner and are associated with increased risk of palmar hyperlinearity; in fact, palmar hyperlinearity is often considered a sign of filaggrin mutations.[35] A recent study of 50 Saudi Arabian children with AD found that 92% had eye findings, including eyelid disease (54%) and keratitis (44%), suspected (16%) or moderate risk (8%) for keratoconus.[36] These findings support the need for regular eye examinations in children with AD. The frequency of keratitis demonstrates that many patients may already have keratitis even without the use of biologic therapy.

ATOPIC COMORBIDITIES

Children with AD have a greater risk of asthma, hay fever, and food allergy, a risk that increases in children with warts.[15] Adults bear the risk of comorbid asthma and hay fever in 8% and 7.5% of patients, respectively. The risk of atopic comorbidities in the setting of AD is sometimes conceptualized as the atopic march, in which cutaneous atopy progresses to systemic allergies and asthma. Mechanistically, percutaneous exposure to food antigens in dust or otherwise in the setting of AD is known to contribute to food allergy development. More formally, this is termed association of AD with the allergen-specific TH2 driven disorders, wherein AD onset and the associated barrier defects promote susceptibility to food allergy and asthma.[37] As some of the comorbidities can overlap in terms of the timing of occurrence, the march may be a cluster for some individuals. Studies that have examined the march/cluster include the Canadian Healthy Infant Longitudinal Development study, a study showing that the presence of AD and sensitization increased asthma risk in young children.[38] A UK study following patients longitudinally showed an increased asthma risk for early-onset AD when checking at age 23 and 44 years.[39] The Avon Longitudinal Study of Parents and Children found all types of AD were associated with asthma especially the persistent type and AD with evidence of the atopic march.[40] The Odense study addressed a cohort of eighth graders with AD and their course of illness. At age 29 years, 50% had persistent AD, 36.3% reported asthma ever, and 60.8% reported ever allergic rhinitis. Additional comorbidities in the allergic or atopic multimorbidities include eosinophilic esophagitis which can be triggered by food allergy and can trigger failure to thrive. This condition can occur at any age.[41] Chronic urticaria is also associated with AD; however, this can be either an allergic or an autoimmune comorbidity. Therefore, laboratory screening for autoimmune thyroid disease may be of benefit to the patient.[42,43] Early-onset and hand eczema were significant risk factors.[44] AD in infancy imparts an allergic risk over a lifetime. Interestingly, the shared importance of IL-4, and to an extent IL-13, in the pathophysiology of these conditions makes drugs impacting IL-4 and IL-13 an important therapeutic benefiting many, most, or all of the allergic comorbidities concurrently. The impact on long-term suppression of IL-4 and IL-13 on the atopic march is unknown but seems promising.[45]

AUTOIMMUNE COMORBIDITIES

In the past 15 years, the association of autoimmune disease with AD was explored in larger series. Alopecia areata (AA) is associated with AD. It was demonstrated that patients with AA and AD are more likely to have extensive hair loss and be refractory to therapy. Further, case reports demonstrate dupilumab has benefit in AD and AA, even demonstrating hair repigmentation.[46,47] Although the association of vitiligo with AD was reported in children under 12 years of age in survey, but not in adults.[47–49] We also have no data on the lifetime impact of AD on course of disease in vitiligo, although AD specifically aggravates the risk of severe disease in AA.[50] We do have data demonstrating overlapping therapeutic benefits for some topical and systemic Janus kinase inhibitors. The current comorbidity guidelines of the AAD for AD acknowledge AA, but not vitiligo, as a common comorbidity.[51]

Although the association with urticaria was addressed under the allergic comorbidities, in fact, some cases are autoimmune, being associated with IgE autoantibody production against the FcER1 receptor. The association of chronic urticaria with AD was made in multiple population-based demographic studies.[42]

Granuloma annulare (GA) is linked to AD in some patients. In a case series of 47 children, 48.9% of children with GA had an atopic condition.[52] Interestingly, there were published case reports of

dupilumab clearing GA, suggesting a shared role for IL-4 and IL-13 in GA and AD.[53,54]

TRAUMATIC COMORBIDITIES

Injuries and fractures have a multifactorial association with AD.[55] Injuries and fractures are more likely to happen in the setting of sleep disturbance and impaired daytime wakefulness, as well as in the setting of reduced bone mineral density (BMD) that can be seen in AD. Although conceptually, oral corticosteroids are a concern for BMD, in fact, one study linked low BMD to cyclosporine usage.[55,56]

ENDOCRINE/METABOLIC COMORBIDITIES

Again, the broad issue of metabolic syndrome and endocrine comorbidities of AD are beyond the scope of this article. However, there is evidence that metabolic syndrome can begin early in life for some AD patients. The authors have found linkage of childhood AD to metabolic syndrome, including increased blood pressure and waist circumference, and non-alcoholic fatty liver disease.[57] Overweight, obesity, and metabolic syndrome linkage to AD appears a particularly high risk in severe AD.[58] The role of adipocytes in inflammation and immune dysregulation was speculated as the reason for association with AD.[59] The recent AAD guidelines discussing comorbidity awareness stated that AD was not associated with diabetes but was linked to obesity, dyslipidemia, hypertension, and CAD.[5] Concerns for nutritional health particularly arise in children with food allergy or eosinophilic esophagitis–related dietary restrictions and linkage to malnutrition was observed.[55]

PSYCHIATRIC COMORBIDITIES

AAD guidelines on comorbidities awareness state that AD is associated with clinician-diagnosed depression, and anxiety, with lower certainty of evidence for suicidality and alcohol abuse. Additionally, attention deficit hyperactivity disorder (ADHD) was linked with low evidence.[5] However, we want to highlight that the neuropsychiatric effects of AD start in infancy with sleep disturbance and irritability associated with sleep disturbances.[60] As children get older, concentration can be impaired with greater sleep disturbance and severe AD being associated with ADHD.[61] ADHD can be associated with anemia, obesity, and headaches in children as well.[61] Preadolescents through adulthood can experience more anxiety and depression, with suicidality being the severe end of the spectrum.[62] All these associations are most common with severe AD.[5]

Comorbid environmental allergy may exacerbate risk of psychiatric comorbidities. In environmental allergies, the immune system overreacts overzealously and inappropriately to allergens in the surroundings. The culprit for these manifestations is that the immune system releases proinflammatory and inflammatory mediators. These same inflammatory cytokine mediators were linked to depression.[63] Research has disclosed that cytokines released in allergic rhinitis can affect monoaminergic neurotransmission and that this may play a role as a risk factor in depression and other mood disorders.[63,64] Depressed individuals were noted to have increased amounts of acute phase proteins, proinflammatory cytokines, chemokines, and cellular adhesion molecules.[63,64] In addition to inflammatory mediators, changes in hormonal levels can contribute to depression and mood disorder. IL-1, IL-6, and tumor necrosis factor alpha are reported to affect corticotrope-releasing hormone which in turn increase adrenocorticotropic hormone and cortisol production via the hypothalamic-pituitary-adrenal pathway and systemic inflammatory markers can precede the appearance of psychiatric disease by a decade.[65–67] Cross-sectional studies and case-control studies showed a relationship between allergic rhinitis and environmental allergies with depression and mood disorders.[68–71]

There are studies where the effect of hormones and mediators are less supportive. These results attribute depression and other mental health sequelae to medications, behavior such as physical and emotional symptoms resulting from the atopic disease manifestations.[72] Exposure to pollen, dust, mold, and even pets can solicit symptoms such as itchy, congested, and runny nose; sneezing; itchy and watery eyes; and other prodromes. Such behavior can stigmatize an individual and disrupt social interactions leading to isolation as well as decrease a person's confidence. Eczema with concomitant unsightly scratching and intractable pruritus can disturb sleep patterns as well as interfere with daily functions. The discomfort of allergy sufferers can result in a negative quality of life which can culminate into anxiety and depression. Allergies impact an individual's well-being, which can interfere with ability to function which for adults is detrimental to work productivity and in children, school performance and scholastic achievements. A link between allergy and suicide was reported.[73,74]

SUMMARY

AD is a multisystem inflammatory disorder beginning in the skin but linking to a series of dominoes falling in the immune system triggering or aggravating tendency to a host of immune and inflammatory events, as well as the long-term outcomes of a lifetime of sleep disturbance. Now that we understand what we need to prevent, interventions can be assessed for their long-term benefits on general health.

CLINICS CARE POINTS

- VINDICATE-P is a mnemonic that captures a large number of the comorbidities of Atopic Dermatitis.
- VINDICATE-P stands for Vascular and cardiovascular, Infections, neoplastic/ neurologic, degeneritive, iatrogenic, congenital, atopy/ autoimmune, traumatic, endocrine/ metabolic, and psychiatric comorbidities.
- Vigilience is needed for early-recognition and control of comorbidites of atopic dermatitis.

DISCLOSURE

J.I. Silverberg has received honoraria as a consultant and/or advisory board member for Abbvie, Alamar, Aldena, Amgen, AObiome, Apollo, Arcutis, Arena, Asana, Aslan, Attovia, BioMX, Biosion, Bodewell, Boehringer-Ingelheim, Bristell-Meyers Squibb, Cara, Castle Biosciences, Celgene, Connect Biopharma, Corevitas, Dermavant, Eli Lilly, FIDE, Galderma, GlaxoSmithKline, Incyte, Inmagene, Invea, Kiniksa, Leo Pharma, Merck, My-Or Diagnostics, Nektar, Novartis, Optum, Pfizer, RAPT, Recludix, Regeneron, Sandoz, Sanofi-Genzyme, Shaperon, TARGET-RWE, Teva, Union, UpToDate; speaker for Abbvie, Eli Lilly, Leo Pharma, Pfizer, Regeneron, Sanofi-Genzyme; institution received grants from Galderma, Incyte, Pfizer. Nanette Silverberg has received honoraria as a consultant, speaker, and/ or advisory board member for Incyte, Leo. Novan, Pfizer, Regeneron, Sanofi-Genzyme, and Verrica Pharmaceuticals.

REFERENCES

1. Marre IR. Infantile eczema. Postgrad Med 1946;22: 190–2.
2. Maciag MC, Phipitanakul W. Preventing the development of asthma: stopping the atopic march. Curr Opin Allergy Clin Immunol 2019;19:161–8.
3. Hanifin JM, Rajka G. Diagnostic features of atopic dermatitis. Acta Derm Venereol 1980;92S:44–7.
4. Dutta A, De A, Das S, et al. A cross-sectional evaluation of the usefulness of the minor features of

hanifin and rajka diagnostic criteria for the diagnosis of atopic dermatitis in the pediatric population. Indian J Dermatol 2021;66:583–90.

5. Davis DMR, Drucker AM, Alikhan A, et al. American Academy of Dermatology Guidelines: Awareness of comorbidities associated with atopic dermatitis in adults. J Am Acad Dermatol 2022;86:1335–6.e18.

6. Available at: https://newsroom.heart.org/news/more-than-half-of-u-s-adults-dont-know-heart-disease-is-leading-cause-of-death-despite-100-year-reign#:~:text=Last%20year%2C%20the%20number%20of,of%20the%20arteries%20(2.6%25. [Accessed 29 January 2024].

7. Silverberg JI. Association between adult atopic dermatitis, cardiovascular disease, and increased heart attacks in three population-based studies. Allergy 2015;70:1300–8.

8. Su VY, Chen TJ, Yeh CM, et al. Atopic dermatitis and risk of ischemic stroke: a nationwide population-based study. Ann Med 2014;46:84–9.

9. Craver AE, Chen GF, Cohen JM. Association between atopic dermatitis and hypertension and hyperlipidemia: A cross-sectional study in the All of Us Research Program. J Am Acad Dermatol 2023; 24. S0190-9622(23)03226-7.

10. Kern C, Ortiz C, Johanis M, et al. Atopic dermatitis and cardiovascular risk in pediatric patients: a systematic review and meta-analysis. J Invest Dermatol 2023. S0022-202X(23)03040-3.

11. Kekki OM, Scheynius A, Poikonen S, et al. Sensitization to Malassezia in children with atopic dermatitis combined with food allergy. Pediatr Allergy Immunol 2013;24:244–9.

12. Silverberg NB. Molluscum contagiosum virus infection can trigger atopic dermatitis disease onset or flare. Cutis 2018;102:191–4.

13. Silverberg JI, Kleiman E, Silverberg NB, et al. Chickenpox in childhood is associated with decreased atopic disorders, IgE,allergic sensitization, and leukocyte subsets. Pediatr Allergy Immunol 2012;23:50–8.

14. Silverberg JI, Norowitz KB, Kleiman E, et al. Association between varicella zoster virus infection and atopic dermatitis in early and late childhood: a case-control study. J AllergyClin Immunol 2010; 126:300–5.

15. Unger L. Kaposi's varicelliform eruption: relation to atopic dermatitis. Ann Allergy 1947;5:426–33.

16. Silverberg JI, Silverberg NB. Childhood atopic dermatitis and warts are associated with increased risk of infection: a US population-based study. J Allergy Clin Immunol 2014;133:1041.

17. Wessels MW, Doekes G, Van Ieperen-Van Kijk AG, et al. IgE antibodies to Pityrosporum ovale in atopic dermatitis. Br J Dermatol 1991;125:227–32.

18. Mathes EF, Oza V, Frieden IJ, et al. "Eczema coxsackium" and unusual cutaneous findings in an enterovirus outbreak. Pediatrics 2013;132:e149–57.

19. Kiiski V, Ukkola-Vuoti L, Vikkula J, et al. Effect of disease severity on comorbid conditions in atopic dermatitis: nationwide registry-based investigation in finnish adults. Acta Derm Venereol 2023;103:adv00882.

20. Ren Z, Silverberg JI. Association of atopic dermatitis with bacterial, fungal, viral, and sexually transmitted skin infections. Dermatitis 2020;31:157–64.

21. Wan J, Shin DB, Syed MN, et al. Malignancy risk in patients with atopic dermatitis: a population-based cohort study. Br J Dermatol 2023;189:53–61.

22. Legendre L, Barnetche T, Mazereeuw-Hautier J, et al. Risk of lymphoma in patients with atopic dermatitis and the role of topical treatment: A systematic review and meta-analysis. J Am Acad Dermatol 2015;72:992–1002.

23. Silverberg JI, Joks R, Durkin HG. Allergic disease is associated with epilepsy in childhood: a US population-based study. Allergy 2014;69:95–103.

24. Fuxench ZCC, Wan J, Wang S, et al. Atopic dermatitis and risk for headache disorders and migraines: a population-based cohort study in children and adults from the UK. Br J Dermatol 2023;190:120–3.

25. Han JH, Lee HJ, Yook HJ, et al. Atopic disorders and their risks of migraine: a nationwide population-based cohort study. Allergy Asthma Immunol Res 2023;15:55–66.

26. Fan R, Leasure AC, Damsky W, et al. Migraine among adults with atopic dermatitis: a cross-sectional study in the All of Us research programme. Clin Exp Dermatol 2023;48:24–6.

27. Yu SH, Drucker AM, Lebwohl M, et al. A systematic review of the safety and efficacy of systemic corticosteroids in atopic dermatitis. J Am Acad Dermatol 2018;78:733–40.

28. Gether L, Storgaard H, Kezic S, et al. Effects of topical corticosteroid versus tacrolimus on insulin sensitivity and bone homeostasis in adults with atopic dermatitis-A randomized controlled study. Allergy 2023;78:1964–79.

29. Kim S, Choi J, Cho MK, et al. Bone mineral density and osteoporosis risk in young adults with atopic dermatitis. Sci Rep 2021;11:24228.

30. Imhof RL, Weaver AL, St Sauver J, et al. Association between topical corticosteroid use and fracture risk among pediatric patients with atopic dermatitis. J Am Acad Dermatol 2022;87:409–11.

31. Mirzakhani H, Al-Garawi A, Weiss ST, et al. Vitamin D and the development of allergic disease: how important is it? Clin Exp Allergy 2015;45:114–25.

32. Reinholz M, Ruzicka T, Schauber J. Vitamin D and its role in allergic disease. Clin Exp Allergy 2012;42: 817–26.

33. Davis DMR, Drucker AM, Alikhan A, et al. Executive summary: Guidelines of care for the management of atopic dermatitis in adults with phototherapy and systemic therapies. J Am Acad Dermatol 2024;90: 342–5.

34. Shetty NS, Lunge S, Sardesai VR, et al. A Cross-Sectional Study Comparing Application of Hanifin and Rajka Criteria in Indian Pediatric Atopic Dermatitis Patients to that of Other Countries. Indian Dermatol Online J 2022;14:32–3.

35. Fukuie T, Yasuoka R, Fujiyama T, et al. Palmar hyperlinearity in early childhood atopic dermatitis is associated with filaggrin mutation and sensitization to egg. Pediatr Dermatol 2019;36:213–21836.

36. Raffa LH, Roblah TM, Balbaid NT, et al. Ocular manifestations of children with atopic dermatitis in Saudi Arabia. Int J Ophthalmol 2023;16:787–93.

37. Paller AS, Spergel JM, Mina-Osorio P, et al. The atopic march and atopic multimorbidity: many trajectories, many pathways. J Allergy Clin Immunol 2019;143:46–55.

38. Tran MM, Lefebvre DL, Dharma C, et al. Predicting the atopic march: results from the Canadian Healthy Infant Longitudinal Development study. J Allergy Clin Immunol 2018;141:601–7.

39. Abo-Zaid G, Sharpe RA, Fleming LE, et al. Association of infant eczema with childhood and adult asthma: analysis of data from the 1958 birth cohort study. Int J Environ Res Publ Health 2018;15:1415.

40. Paternoster L, Savenije OEM, Heron J, et al. Identification of atopic dermatitis subgroups in children from 2 longitudinal birth cohorts. J Allergy Clin Immunol 2018;141:964–71.

41. Muir A, Falk GW. Eosinophilic esophagitis: a review. JAMA 2021;326:1310–8.

42. Chiu HY, Muo CH, Sung FC. Associations of chronic urticaria with atopic and autoimmune comorbidities: a nationwide population-based study. Int J Dermatol 2018;57:822–9.

43. Magen E, Chikovani T, Waitman DA, et al. Association of alopecia areata with atopic dermatitis and chronic spontaneous urticaria. Allergy Asthma Proc 2018;39:96–102.

44. Mortz CG, Andersen KE, Dellgren C, et al. Atopic dermatitis from adolescence to adulthood in the TOACS cohort: prevalence, persistence and comorbidities. Allergy 2015;70:836–45.

45. Cai L, Wei Y, Zhao M, et al. Case report: Dupilumab therapy for alopecia areata in a 4-year-old patient resistant to baricitinib. Front Med 2023;10:1253795.

46. Yan X, Tayier M, Cheang ST, et al. Hair repigmentation and regrowth in a dupilumab-treated paediatric patient with alopecia areata and atopic dermatitis: a case report. Ther Adv Chronic Dis 2023;14. 20406223231191049.

47. Fenner J, Silverberg NB. Skin diseases associated with atopic dermatitis. Clin Dermatol 2018;36:631–40.

48. Mohan GC, Silverberg JI. Association of vitiligo and alopecia areata with atopic dermatitis: a systematic review and meta-analysis. JAMA Dermatol 2015;151:522–8.

49. Silverberg JI, Silverberg NB. Association between vitiligo and atopic disorders: a pilot study. JAMA Dermatol 2013;149:983–6.

50. Ezzedine K, Diallo A, Léauté-Labrèze C, et al. Pre- vs. post-pubertal onset of vitiligo: multivariate analysis indicates atopic diathesis association in pre-pubertal onset vitiligo. Br J Dermatol 2012;167:490–5.

51. Davis DMR, Drucker AM, Alikhan A, et al. American Academy of Dermatology Guidelines: Awareness of comorbidities associated with atopic dermatitis in adults. J Am Acad Dermatol 2022;86:1335–6.

52. Cruz SA, Stein SL. The clinical presentation and co-morbidities associated with granuloma annulare in the pediatric population: a retrospective study. Skinmed 2022;20:24–8.

53. Song EJ, Bezecny J, Farrer S. Recalcitrant generalized granuloma annulare treated successfully with dupilumab. JAAD Case Rep 2020;7:1–2.

54. Song X, Chen Z, Zhao Z, et al. Treatment of generalized granuloma annulare with dupilumab. J Dermatol Treat 2023;34:2186158.

55. Silverberg JI. Selected comorbidities of atopic dermatitis: Atopy, neuropsychiatric, and musculoskeletal disorders. Clin Dermatol 2017;35:360–6.

56. Silverberg JI. Association between childhood atopic dermatitis, malnutrition, and low bone mineral density: A US population-based study. Pediatr Allergy Immunol 2015;26:54–61.

57. Reddy P, Mahajan R, Mehta H, et al. Increased prevalence of metabolic syndrome and non-alcoholic fatty liver disease in children with atopic dermatitis: A case-control study from northern India. Pediatr Dermatol 2024. https://doi.org/10.1111/pde.15502. Epub ahead of print.

58. Gonzalez-Uribe V, Vidaurri-de la Cruz H, Gomez-Nuñez A, et al. Comorbidities & burden of disease in atopic dermatitis. Asian Pac J Allergy Immunol 2023;41:97–105.

59. De Simoni E, Rizzetto G, Molinelli E, et al. Metabolic comorbidities in pediatric atopic dermatitis: a narrative review. Life 2022;13:2.

60. Guo Y, Zhang H, Liu Q, et al. Phenotypic analysis of atopic dermatitis in children aged 1-12 months: elaboration of novel diagnostic criteria for infants in China and estimation of prevalence. J Eur Acad Dermatol Venereol 2019;33:1569–76.

61. Strom MA, Fishbein AB, Paller AS, et al. Association between atopic dermatitis and attention deficit hyperactivity disorder in U.S. children and adults. Br J Dermatol 2016;175:920–9.

62. Kamal K, Xiang DH, Young K, et al. Comorbid psychiatric disease significantly mediates increased rates of alcohol use disorder among patients with inflammatory and pigmentary skin disorders: a case-control study in the All of Us Research Program. Arch Dermatol Res 2024;316:79.

63. Raison CL, Capuron L, Miller AH. Cytokines sing the blues: inflammation and the pathogenesis of depression. Trends Immunol 2006;27:24–31.
64. Oh H, Koyanagi A, DeVylder JE, et al. Seasonal allergies and psychiatric disorders in the United States. Int J Environ Res Publ Health 2018;15:1965.
65. Leffa DT, Caye A, Santos I, et al. Attention-deficit/hyperactivity disorder has a state-dependent association with asthma: The role of systemic inflammation in a population-based birth cohort followed from childhood to adulthood. Brain Behav Immun 2021; 97:239–49.
66. Tamm S, Cervenka S, Forsberg A, et al. Evidence of fatigue, disordered sleep and peripheral inflammation, but not increased brain TSPO expression, in seasonal allergy: A [11C]PBR28 PET study. Brain Behav Immun 2018;68:146–57.
67. Khandaker GM, Zammit S, Lewis G, et al. A population-based study of atopic disorders and inflammatory markers in childhood before psychotic experiences in adolescence. Schizophr Res 2014; 152:139–45.
68. Chen MH, Su TP, Chen YS, et al. Allergic rhinitis in adolescence increases the risk of depression in later life: A nationwide population-based prospective cohort study. J Affect Disord 2013;145:49–53.
69. Kim DH, Han K, Kim SW. Relationship between allergic rhinitis and mental health in the general Korean adult population. Allergy Asthma Immunol. Res 2016;8:49–54.
70. Postolache TT, Lapidus M, Sander ER, et al. Changes in allergy symptoms and depression scores are positively correlated in patients with recurrent mood disorders exposed to seasonal peaks in aeroallergens. Sci World J 2007;7: 1968–77.
71. Patten SB, Williams JV. Self-reported allergies and their relationship to several Axis I disorders in a community sample. Int J Psychiatr Med 2007;37: 11–22.
72. Glaus J, Vandeleur CL, von Känel R, et al. Associations between mood, anxiety or substance use disorders and inflammatory markers after adjustment for multiple covariates in a population-based study. J Psychiatr Res 2014;58:36–45.
73. Qin P, Mortensen PB, Waltoft BL, et al. Allergy is associated with suicide completion with a possible mediating role of mood disorder—A population-based study. Allergy 2011;66:658–64.
74. Stickley A, Ng CFS, Konishi S, et al. Airborne pollen and suicide mortality in Tokyo, 2001–2011. Environ Res 2017;155:134–40.

Topical Therapy for Atopic Dermatitis

What is New and the New Paradigm

Maria Gnarra Buethe, MD, PhD[a,b,1], Caitlyn Kellogg, MD[a,b,2],
Young Joon Seo, MD[a,b,c,3], Carrie Vuong, MD[a,b,4],
Lawrence F. Eichenfield, MD[a,b,d],*

KEYWORDS

• Atopic dermatitis • Topicals • Ruxolitinib • Roflumilast • Crisaborole • Tapinarof

KEY POINTS

• Ruxolitinib 1.5% cream is a topical Janus kinase 1 (JAK1)/JAK2 inhibitor approved for mild-to-moderate atopic dermatitis (AD) in patients aged 12+ years. Efficacy data show superiority to triamcinolone 0.1% cream and good disease control up to 1 year.
• Roflumilast cream emerges as a novel and effective daily topical PDE-4 inhibitor for AD, presenting a promising treatment option that has demonstrated significant symptom relief and safety profile.
• Once-daily application of crisaborole, 2% ointment could be a potential long-term maintenance treatment option in children and adult patients with mild-to-moderate AD.
• Topical tapinarof is an aryl hydrocarbon receptor agonist currently under investigation for the treatment of AD, and data thus far demonstrate its efficacy and safety.
• New nonsteroidal topical agents expand our armamentarium in achieving effective long-term disease control in AD, filling a previously unmet need for therapies that balance efficacy with limited long-term adverse effects.

INTRODUCTION

Atopic dermatitis (AD) is a chronic, inflammatory skin disease with the prevalence of 11.3% to 12.7% in children and 6.9% to 7.6% in adults in the United States.[1] It is characterized by a T-helper type 2 (Th2) immune response with upregulation of proinflammatory cytokines including interleukin (IL)-4, IL-5, IL-13, IL-31, and the Janus kinase-signal transducer and activator of transcription (JAK-STAT) signaling pathway.[2] Also central to the pathogenesis of AD is dysfunction of the skin barrier characterized by lower expression of epidermal protein-coding genes such as filaggrin (FLG) and loricrin (LOR), alterations in epidermal lipids, and increased epidermal water loss.[3,4]

Among the Food and Drug Administration (FDA)-approved therapies for AD, topical corticosteroids (TCSs) are the most commonly utilized[5]; however, side effects of long-term use including atrophy, striae, rosacea, perioral dermatitis, acne and purpura, and steroid phobia among patients leads to

a Division of Pediatric and Adolescent Dermatology, Rady Children's Hospital San Diego, San Diego, CA, USA;
b Department of Dermatology, University of California San Diego School of Medicine, La Jolla, CA, USA;
c Department of Dermatology, Chungnam National University College of Medicine, Daejeon, Korea;
d Department of Pediatrics, University of California San Diego School of Medicine, La Jolla, CA, USA
1 Present address: 2683 Via de la Valle, Suite G #210, Del Mar, CA 92014.
2 Present address: 6501 Forum Street, San Diego, CA 92111.
3 Present address: 11232 Vista Sorrento Parkway, M210, San Diego, CA 92130.
4 Present address: 3071 Sunset Canyon Drive, San Diego, CA 92117.
* Corresponding author. 3020 Children's Way, Mail Code 5092, San Diego, CA 92123.
E-mail address: leichenfield@rchsd.org

Dermatol Clin 42 (2024) 569–575
https://doi.org/10.1016/j.det.2024.05.001

medication nonadherence.[6,7] In addition, there are many gaps in research on TCSs including comparative data between TCS and nonsteroidal topical medications, as well as data on utilization of TCSs in flare prevention and cost-efficacy.[5] Topical calcineurin inhibitors (TCIs) have been recommended as a nonsteroidal alternative to TCSs and are FDA-approved for patients aged 2 years and above.[5] As research continues to provide further insight into the pathogenesis of AD, new topical nonsteroidal medications are increasingly being implemented in AD care. This review provides an update on recent safety and efficacy data, including Investigator's Global Assessment (IGA), Eczema Area and Severity Index (EASI), and itch numerical rating scale score (NRS4), on the novel topical nonsteroidal medications currently approved by the FDA including, ruxolitinib, PDE-4 inhibitors, and tapinarof, which is currently under investigation for the treatment of AD.

RUXOLITINIB

Ruxolitinib 1.5% cream (Opzelura, Incyte, Wilmington, DE) received FDA approval in September 2021 for short-term (up to 8 weeks) and noncontinuous chronic treatment of mild-to-moderate (IGA score of 2 to 3) AD in nonimmunocompromised patients aged 12 years and older.[8] Ruxolitinib works by inhibiting the JAK-STAT, specifically JAK1 and JAK2.[9] The JAK-STAT pathway plays a pivotal role in the pathogenesis of AD as it is responsible for the recruitment of keratinocytes, immune cells, and peripheral sensory neurons thus propagating pruritus and inflammation.[10] All JAK inhibitors (JAKis) carry black box warnings, referential to data of pan-JAKi tofacitinib in patients aged over 50 years, and at least one cardiovascular risk factor (thus quite a different study population from the usually younger and healthier patients with AD is affected). This includes serious infections, mortality, malignancies (eg, lymphoma), major adverse cardiovascular events (MACEs), and thrombosis.[11]

In maximal-use application studies in adolescents and adults with greater than 25% body surface area (BSA) AD involvement, the mean steady-state ruxolitinib plasma concentration was consistently below the half-maximal inhibitory concentration of JAK-mediated myelosuppression.[12] Pharmacokinetic studies in a phase II and phase III 3 double-blind, vehicle-controlled studies in patients with AD showed that the application of topical 1.5% cream to up to 20% BSA and 60 g per week is not expected to lead to systemic plasma concentrations associated with adverse effects that may be commonly associated with oral JAKis.[13] The most common adverse event (AE) was nasopharyngitis, which,

despite not occurring in most patients, was higher in the ruxolitinib compared to the placebo group.

Phase III, randomized, double-blinded studies (TRuE-AD) have shown how topical ruxolitinib achieved the primary endpoint of an IGA score of 0 to 1 and 2 or greater grade improvement from baseline at week 8 compared with placebo. There have only been a limited number of studies comparing the newer nonsteroid anti-inflammatory agents to topical steroids. However, the Phase II trial (TRuE-AD1) compared twice daily application of topical ruxolitinib to triamcinolone cream 0.1%. After 4 weeks, ruxolitinib showed superiority in several endpoints compared to triamcinolone including IGA clear/almost clear (38% vs 25.5%), EASI-75 (56% vs 47.1%), EASI-90 (26% vs 14.7%) and NRS4-point itch reduction (62.5% vs 32.3%). Impressively, itch relief occurred as fast as 2 days after the first application.[14,15]

Topical ruxolitinib also showed good disease control in open extension studies up to 1 year with an IGA score of 0 or 1 in 74% to 78% of patients at week 52 and 1% to 2% BSA,[16] a dataset that was not available at the time of the American Academy of Dermatology (AAD) guidelines for topical therapy in adults.[5] A recent study (TRUE AD-3) aimed to assess the safety, pharmacokinetics, and efficacy of 0.75% to 1.5% ruxolitinib cream in children and adolescents (2–<12 years) with AD. After twice-daily application for 28 days, ruxolitinib cream showed no serious treatment-emergent AEs. Additionally, no effect on blood counts or bone biomarkers were observed.[17] The study met its primary endpoint and showed significantly more patients treated with ruxolitinib cream 0.75% and 1.5% achieved IGA 0 (clear) or 1 (almost clear) with at least a 2 point improvement from baseline at week 8, compared to vehicles. Safety data was consistent with what was observed in adults, with low rates of discontinuation.[18]

PDE-4 INHIBITORS

PDE-4 is an intracellular enzyme mainly present in immune, epithelial, and brain cells that regulates inflammation and epithelial integrity by degrading cyclic adenosine monophosphate.[19] PDE-4 inhibition mediates inflammatory cytokines and has been utilized in various forms for respiratory diseases, cutaneous psoriasis, psoriatic arthritis, and AD.[20,21]

Roflumilast

Topical roflumilast, is a novel PDE-4 inhibitor that has shown efficacy in managing psoriasis, AD, and seborrheic dermatitis, with respective formulations tailored to each condition.[22–24] Specifically, the 0.3% cream formulation is FDA-approved for psoriasis treatment in patients aged 6 years and older, while the 0.3% foam is sanctioned for those aged 9 years and above with seborrheic dermatitis. In the development program for AD, roflumilast 0.15% cream has successfully demonstrated its therapeutic potential in 2 phase III trials (INTEGU-MENT-1: NCT04773587[25] and INTEGUMENT-2: NCT04773600[26]). In the clinical studies, patient eligibility was determined by being aged 6 years or older, having a validated investigator global assessment (vIGA)-AD score of 2 or 3, a BSA involvement of 3 or more, and an EASI score of 5 or greater. Significantly higher percentage (31.3%) of patients achieved vIGA-AD success, defined as "Clear" or "Almost Clear" skin plus a 2 grade improvement from baseline. Roflumilast cream significantly reduced EASI scores, with 377 out of 884 patients (42.7%) of patients achieving 75% reductions in EASI scores by the end of the study period. Improvements in itch were noted as early as 24 hours after the first application of roflu-milast cream, and these improvements were more significant than those observed with the vehicle. Roflumilast cream was well tolerated with low inci-dence of application site AEs. Tolerability was high, with most participants reporting minimal to no discomfort at the application site.

These findings are corroborated by another phase III trial of 0.05% roflumilast cream (INTEGU-MENT-PED: NCT04845620)[27] that displayed roflu-milast's effectiveness and safety in a pediatric cohort aged 2 to 5 years. The study demonstrated that roflumilast was well tolerated and effective, showing significant improvements in AD symp-toms over 4 weeks. Marked improvement in vIGA-AD scores with significant differences from the vehicle were recorded, appearing as early as week 1. A total of 154 out of 436 patients (35.3%) achieved a vIGA-AD status of clear or almost clear at week 4. Additionally, 172 out of 436 patients (39.4%) reached EASI-75. Pruritus, assessed daily, also showed significant improve-ments from baseline, which were noticeable within 24 hours after the first application of the cream. The treatment was generally safe with low inci-dence of AEs, none of which were serious or led to discontinuation in more than a few cases. This aligns with the known safety profile of roflumilast in previous studies on different age groups and conditions. The study's results are promising, sug-gesting that roflumilast cream 0.05% could be a valuable nonsteroidal treatment option for young children aged 2 to 5 years with AD.

Longer term studies of roflumilast are currently underway to further evaluate its sustained efficacy and safety.

Crisaborole

Crisaborole, 2% ointment, is a PDE-4 inhibitor that has been approved by the FDA for the treatment of mild-to-moderate AD in patients aged as young as 3 months.[28,29]

Recently, the CrisADe CONTROL study investi-gated the long-term efficacy and safety of crisabor-ole 2% ointment, as a maintenance treatment of AD (NCT04040192).[30] This study evaluated how effec-tive and safe long-term treatment with once daily crisaborole was compared with a vehicle. Patients who showed high levels of improvement with twice-daily crisaborole during an 8 week run-in period (clear/almost clear [0–1 with a ≥2 grade improve-ment in IGA] and ≥50% EASI improvement) were randomized to receive either crisaborole or vehicle once daily for 52 weeks. The study included 497 pa-tients initially, with 270 successfully completing the run-in period and being randomized for the mainte-nance phase. The median time to the first flare was significantly longer for patients treated with crisa-borole (111 days) compared to those receiving the vehicle (30 days). Patients treated with crisa-borole experienced more flare-free days on average (234 days) than those treated with the vehicle (199.4 days) and had fewer flares (average of 0.95 flares) compared to those on the vehicle (average of 1.36 flares). Crisaborole was well toler-ated with no new or unexpected safety findings re-ported. These results indicate that once-daily treatment with crisaborole could be a potential long-term maintenance treatment option in chil-dren and adults with mild-to-moderate AD.

TAPINAROF

Topical tapinarof 1% (VTAMA, Dermavant Sci-ences, Inc., Morrisville, NC) (TAP1%) is an aryl hy-drocarbon receptor (AhR) agonist currently approved for the treatment of plaque psoriasis in adults and under investigation for the treatment of AD.[1,2] The AhR is a ligand-activated transcription factor expressed in keratinocytes and a variety of immune cells.[31–33] AhR activity promotes the integ-rity of the skin barrier and regulates skin homeosta-sis[31]; it has been shown to upregulate skin barrier components including LOR, involucrin, FLG, hor-nerin, and ceramide lipids, attenuate the generation and survival of resident memory T cells, and decrease Th2 proinflammatory cytokines including IL-4, IL-5, IL-13, and IL-31.[34–36] A recent study uti-lizing human immortalized keratinocytes treated with AhR ligands demonstrated Tapinarof's ability to attenuate the expression of multiple IL-13-dependent, AD-related genes including eosinophil chemoattractant CCL26 (eotaxin-3).[37] In addition,

AhR may function through antioxidant activity through nuclear factor erythroid 2-related factor (Nrf2)-mediated pathways.[34,35]

A phase IIa, open-label, maximum-use trial of tapinarof cream among patients aged 2 to 17 years with vIGA for AD score of 3 or greater and 25% or greater BSA involvement (12–17 years) or 35% or greater involvement showed that tapinarof was well tolerated with a consistent pharmacokinetic profile and performance among all ages and disease states, low incidence of AEs with no significant systemic AEs, no contact dermatitis, and minimal to no systemic exposure under maximal use conditions for patients with up to 90% BSA affected.[38] ADORING 1 and 2 were 2 identical recent phase III clinical trials including 407 (ADORING 1) and 406 (ADORING 2) adult and pediatric patients aged 2 years or older with vIGA-AD 3 or greater, 5% to 35% BSA, and EASI 6 or greater. After 8 weeks, these trials demonstrated significant reductions in vIGA (45% TAP1% vs 14% vehicle and 46% TAP1% vs 18% vehicle in ADORING 1 and 2, respectively, achieved vIGA-AD success, defined as vIGA-AD 0 or 1 with 2 point or greater improvement from baseline, both $P < .0001$), EASI 75 (56% TAP1% vs 23% vehicle and 59% TAP1% vs 21% vehicle in ADORING 1 and 2, respectively, both $P < .0001$), and 4 point reduction or greater in PP-NRS (56% TAP1% vs 34% placebo [$P = .0366$] and 53% TAP1% vs 24% vehicle [$P = .0015$] in ADORING 1 and 2, respectively).[39] Safety data demonstrated that AEs were mild to moderate and the discontinuation rate was decreased compared to vehicle (ADORING 1: 1.9% TAP1% vs 3.6% vehicle; ADORING 2: 1.5% VTMA vs 3.0% vehicle).[39]

In addition, tapinarof treatment resulted in meaningful improvements in patient-reported outcomes including dermatology life quality index (DLQI), children's dermatology life quality index (CDLQI), infants' dermatitis quality of life index (IDQOL), and patient-oriented eczema measure (POEM) (Simpson AAD presentation).[40] The most common AEs in phase III trials were "follicular events," observed in approximately 9% to 10% of patients with AD on tapinarof and headache. Interim analysis of ADORING 3, a 48 week open-label, long-term extension study among 711 patients with vIGA-AD 3 or greater, demonstrated safety of tapinarof and continued improvements in efficacy beyond 8 weeks (Adoring 3 press release).[39,41]

PARADIGM: NOVEL AND TRADITIONAL TOPICALS IN REGIMENS OF CARE

Topical anti-inflammatories remain a mainstay in the management of pediatric AD. Best practices in prescribing topical agents include delineation of both flare and maintenance regimens and adequate explanation of appropriate volumes to use for each scenario. Especially in the pediatric population, fear of side effects of topical agents, especially topical steroids, as well as a lack of understanding of appropriate volumes to apply for different body sizes and disease extent can contribute to undertreatment and poor adherence. The principle of suggesting appropriate quantities of topical medication to use for varying surface area and body size has been termed "volumetric prescriptions."[42] A standardized tool facilitating volumetric prescriptions was developed in a support program for pediatricians to improve care of AD. This "topical medication volume calculator" is integrated into the electronic health record and estimates the volume (in grams) of topical medications to be used in a typical several-week tapered regimen based on patient age and BSA involvement. This was shown to improve provider management of pediatric AD.[42]

Though in most studies novel topical agents are employed as monotherapy and compared to vehicle as part of the drug approval process, in clinical practice, these therapies will likely be utilized in multiagent regimens of care, which may include traditional emollients, good bathing practices, traditional topical steroids, calcineurin inhibitors, and newer nonsteroid anti-inflammatory agents.

Recent guidelines from prominent US and international groups (eg, American Academy of Dermatology, Consensus-based European Guidelines, and American Academy of Allergy, Asthma and Immunology) vary in recommendations for the use of topical therapies for AD and are without specific algorithms for the use of different agents in regimens of care. Commonalties among most of the guidelines are the use of moisturizers as a core aspect of treatment, recognition of topical steroids of varying strengths as a mainstay of therapy, and the use of nonsteroid prescription agents as an alternative to TCS for AD that is refractory to moisturizers, either as reactive therapy for signs and/or symptoms of AD, or as proactive therapy. Factors that can influence selection of topical agents include disease severity, extent, regional anatomy, response to prior therapies, disease course, tolerance to medications, patient and caregiver preference, as well as cost and access.

We propose that providers establish an expectation of long-term disease control, striving for minimal signs of AD, minimal itch, and minimal sleep disturbance. A standard paradigm should be initiation of therapeutic regimens stressing "good skin care" with culturally-accepted bathing and moisturization practices and use of TCSs generally as first-line anti-inflammatory agents for AD unresponsive to general measures, with TCIs (pimecrolimus and tacrolimus), PDE-4 inhibitors (crisaborole and roflumilast), topical JAKis (ruxolitinib), or tapinarof as alternative agents to be considered, subject to drug approval, age or BSA restrictions, as well as cost and access considerations. Beyond acute disease control, intermittent use of TCS or the above nonsteroid agents may be used either "as needed," or in proactive regimens. A recent European study aimed to compare the effects of proactive treatment with tacrolimus ointment and mometasone furoate on the epidermal barrier structure and ceramide levels of patients with AD, showed superiority of TCI.[43]

While there is burden associated with topical regimens for patients and families in terms of time spent applying medicines, cost, and side effects, regimens incorporating new nonsteroidal agents (the PDE-4 inhibitors crisaborole or roflumilast, aryl-hydrocarbon receptor agonist tapinarof, and topical JAKi ruxolitinib) along with TCIs present a paradigm shift in terms of high efficacy in improving inflammation, itch, and barrier function, while limiting the adverse effects associated with long-term use of TCSs. The newer nonsteroid agents expand our armamentarium to achieve effective long-term disease control in AD, either with regimens of care relying on topical medications or together with systemic agents.

CLINICS CARE POINTS

- Evolving non-steroidal topical agents for atopic dermatitis include JAK-inhibitors, PDE-4 inhibitors and an aryl hydrocarbon receptor agonist, all of which can be useful as anti-inflammatory agents.
- Topical ruxolitinib has been studied utilizing a maximum application useage recommendation of no more than 20% body surface area application.
- "Volumetric presribing," setting expectations of volume of application of a topical agent to use over a period of time, may improve outcomes of AD care.

DISCLOSURE

L.F. Eichenfield has served as a consultant, speaker, advisory board member, or investigator for AbbVie, Amgen, Apogee, Arcutis, Aslan, Attovia, Bristol-Myers Squibb, Castle Biosciences, Dermavant, Eli Lilly, Forte, Galderma, Incyte, Janssen, Johnson & Johnson, LEO Pharma, Novartis, Ortho Dermatologics, Pfizer, Regeneron, Sanofi-Genzyme, Target RWE and UCB. M.G. Buethe, C. Kellogg, Y.J. Seo, and C. Vuong have nothing to disclose.

FUNDING

This worked was partially funded by the Rady/University of California San Diego Eczema and Inflammatory Skin Disease Center.

REFERENCES

1. Silverberg JI. Public Health Burden and Epidemiology of Atopic Dermatitis. Dermatol Clin 2017; 35(3):283–9.
2. Fania L, Moretta G, Antonelli F, et al. Multiple Roles for Cytokines in Atopic Dermatitis: From Pathogenic Mediators to Endotype-Specific Biomarkers to Therapeutic Targets. Int J Mol Sci 2022;23(5):2684.
3. Baurecht H, Rühlemann MC, Rodr´guez E, et al. Epidermal lipid composition, barrier integrity, and eczematous inflammation are associated with skin microbiome configuration. J Allergy Clin Immunol 2018;141(5):1668–76.e16.
4. Tsakok T, Woolf R, Smith CH, et al. Atopic dermatitis: the skin barrier and beyond. Br J Dermatol 2019; 180(3):464–74.
5. Sidbury R, Alikhan A, Bercovitch L, et al. Guidelines of care for the management of atopic dermatitis in adults with topical therapies. J Am Acad Dermatol 2023;89(1):e1–20.
6. Hengge UR, Ruzicka T, Schwartz RA, et al. Adverse effects of topical glucocorticosteroids. J Am Acad Dermatol 2006;54(1):1–15.
7. Fitzmaurice W, Silverberg NB. Systematic Review of Steroid Phobia in Atopic Dermatitis. Dermatitis® 2024;derm.2023.0213.
8. Prescribing Information for Opzelura (Ruxolitinib) Cream 1.5%. 2023. Available at: https://www.opzelura.com/prescribing-information.pdf.
9. Chovatiya R, Paller AS. JAK inhibitors in the treatment of atopic dermatitis. J Allergy Clin Immunol 2021;148(4):927–40.
10. Bao L, Zhang H, Chan LS. The involvement of the JAK-STAT signaling pathway in chronic inflammatory skin disease atopic dermatitis. JAK-STAT 2013;2(3): e24137.
11. Ireland PA, Jansson N, Spencer SKR, et al. Short-Term Cardiovascular Complications in Dermatology Patients Receiving JAK-STAT Inhibitors: A Meta-Analysis of Randomized Clinical Trials. JAMA Dermatol 2024;160(3):281.
12. Bissonnette R, Call RS, Raoof T, et al. A Maximum-Use Trial of Ruxolitinib Cream in Adolescents and Adults with Atopic Dermatitis. Am J Clin Dermatol 2022;23(3):355–64.

13. Gong X, Chen X, Kuligowski ME, et al. Pharmacokinetics of Ruxolitinib in Patients with Atopic Dermatitis Treated With Ruxolitinib Cream: Data from Phase II and III Studies. Am J Clin Dermatol 2021; 22(4):555–66.

14. Kim BS, Howell MD, Sun K, et al. Treatment of atopic dermatitis with ruxolitinib cream (JAK1/JAK2 inhibitor) or triamcinolone cream. J Allergy Clin Immunol 2020;145(2):572–82.

15. Papp K, Szepietowski JC, Kircik L, et al. Efficacy and safety of ruxolitinib cream for the treatment of atopic dermatitis: Results from 2 phase 3, randomized, double-blind studies. J Am Acad Dermatol 2021;85(4):863–72.

16. Papp K, Szepietowski JC, Kircik L, et al. Long-term safety and disease control with ruxolitinib cream in atopic dermatitis: Results from two phase 3 studies. J Am Acad Dermatol 2023;88(5):1008–16.

17. Leung DYM, Paller AS, Zaenglein AL, et al. Safety, pharmacokinetics, and efficacy of ruxolitinib cream in children and adolescents with atopic dermatitis. Ann Allergy Asthma Immunol 2023;130(4):500–7.e3.

18. Soong W, Zaenglein A, Tollefson M, et al. Efficacy and Safety of Ruxolitinib Cream Among Children With Atopic Dermatitis Aged 2 to 6 Years and 7 to <12 Years: Results from a Phase 3 Double-Blind Vehicle-Controlled Study. J Allergy Clin Immunol 2024;153(2):AB1.

19. Li H, Zuo J, Tang W. Phosphodiesterase-4 Inhibitors for the Treatment of Inflammatory Diseases. Front Pharmacol 2018;9:1048.

20. Schafer PH, Truzzi F, Parton A, et al. Phosphodiesterase 4 in inflammatory diseases: Effects of apremilast in psoriatic blood and in dermal myofibroblasts through the PDE4/CD271 complex. Cell Signal 2016;28(7):753–63.

21. Zebda R, Paller AS. Phosphodiesterase 4 inhibitors. J Am Acad Dermatol 2018;78(3):S43–52.

22. Lebwohl MG, Kircik LH, Moore AY, et al. Effect of Roflumilast Cream vs Vehicle Cream on Chronic Plaque Psoriasis: The DERMIS-1 and DERMIS-2 Randomized Clinical Trials. JAMA 2022;328(11):1073.

23. Gooderham M, Kircik L, Zirwas M, et al. The Safety and Efficacy of Roflumilast Cream 0.15% and 0.05% in Patients With Atopic Dermatitis: Randomized, Double-Blind, Phase 2 Proof of Concept Study. J Drugs Dermatol JDD 2023;22(2):139–47.

24. Blauvelt A, Draelos ZD, Stein Gold L, et al. Roflumilast foam 0.3% for adolescent and adult patients with seborrheic dermatitis: A randomized, double-blinded, vehicle-controlled, phase 3 trial. J Am Acad Dermatol 2024;90(5):986–93.

25. Clinicaltrials.gov. Trial of PDE4 Inhibition With Roflumilast for the Management of Atopic Dermatitis (INTEGU-MENT-I). 2023. Available at: https://clinicaltrials.gov/study/NCT04773600?cond=NCT04773600&rank=1.

26. Clinicaltrials.gov. Trial of PDE4 Inhibition With Roflumilast for the Management of Atopic Dermatitis (INTEGUMENT-II). 2023. Available at: https://clinicaltrials.gov/study/NCT04773600?cond=NCT04773600&rank=1.

27. Clinicaltrials.gov. Trial of PDE4 Inhibition With Roflumilast for the Management of Atopic Dermatitis (Integument-PED). 2023. Available at: https://clinicaltrials.gov/study/NCT04845620?cond=NCT04845620&rank=1.

28. U.S. Food and Drug Administration. FDA Approves Eucrisa for Eczema. 2016. Available at: https://www.fda.gov/news-events/press-announcements/fda-approves-eucrisa-eczema.

29. U.S. Food and Drug Administration. Eucrisa Prescribing Information. 2020. Available at: https://www.accessdata.fda.gov/drugsatfda_docs/label/2020/207695s007s009s010lbl.pdf.

30. A Study to Evaluate Long-Term Maintenance Treatment With Once Daily Crisaborole Ointment 2% in Pediatric and Adult Participants With Mild-to-Moderate Atopic Dermatitis. 2023. Available at: https://clinicaltrials.gov/study/NCT04040192?cond=NCT04040192&rank=1.

31. Bissonnette R, Stein Gold L, Rubenstein DS, et al. Tapinarof in the treatment of psoriasis: A review of the unique mechanism of action of a novel therapeutic aryl hydrocarbon receptor–modulating agent. J Am Acad Dermatol 2021;84(4):1059–67.

32. Esser C, Rannug A. The Aryl Hydrocarbon Receptor in Barrier Organ Physiology, Immunology, and Toxicology. In: Ma Q, editor. Pharmacol Rev 2015;67(2):259–79.

33. Sutter CH, Olesen KM, Bhuju J, et al. AHR Regulates Metabolic Reprogramming to Promote SIRT1-Dependent Keratinocyte Differentiation. J Invest Dermatol 2019;139(4):818–26.

34. Smith SH, Jayawickreme C, Rickard DJ, et al. Tapinarof Is a Natural AhR Agonist that Resolves Skin Inflammation in Mice and Humans. J Invest Dermatol 2017;137(10):2110–9.

35. Kleinman E, Laborada J, Metterle L, et al. What's New in Topicals for Atopic Dermatitis? Am J Clin Dermatol 2022;23(5):595–603.

36. Mooney N, Teague JE, Gehad AE, et al. Tapinarof Inhibits the Formation, Cytokine Production, and Persistence of Resident Memory T Cells In Vitro. J of Skin 2023;7(2):s194.

37. Proper SP, Dwyer AT, Appiagyei A, et al. Aryl hydrocarbon receptor and IL-13 signaling crosstalk in human keratinocytes and atopic dermatitis. Front Allergy 2024;5:1323405.

38. Dermavant Announces Positive Data from the ADORING Phase 3 Development Program in Atopic Dermatitis with VTAMA® (Tapinarof) Cream, 1% in Adults and Children as Young as 2 Years Old. 2024. Available at: https://dermavant.com/dermavant-announces-positive-data-from-the-adoring-phase-3-development-program-in-atopic-dermatitis-with-vtama-tapinarof-cream-1-in-adults-and-children-as-young-as-2-years-old/.

39. Silverberg JI, Eichenfield LF, Hebert AA, et al. 514 - Tapinarof cream 1% once daily: significant efficacy in the treatment of atopic dermatitis in two pivotal phase 3 trials in adults and children down to 2 years of age. Br J Dermatol 2024;190(Supplement_2): ii17–8.

40. Simpson E, Hebert A, Sofen H, et al. Tapinarof Cream 1% Once Daily in Adults and Children Down to 2 Years of Age with Moderate to Severe Atopic Dermatitis in Two Phase 3 Trials: Patient reported Outcomes. Presented at: March 8, 2024; American Academy of Dermatology (AAD) Congress, San Diego, California.

41. Available at: https://dermavant.com/dermavant-announces-positive-data-from-the-adoring-phase-3-development-program-in-atopic-dermatitis-with-vtama-tapinarof-cream-1-in-adults-and-children-as-young-as-2-years-old/.

42. Lee SS, Kaushik A, Natsis N, et al. A multimodal initiative improves general pediatric provider management of atopic dermatitis in children: A prospective interventional study. J Am Acad Dermatol 2023; 89(5):1041–4.

43. Dähnhardt D, Bastian M, Dähnhardt-Pfeiffer S, et al. Comparing the effects of proactive treatment with tacrolimus ointment and mometasone furoate on the epidermal barrier structure and ceramide levels of patients with atopic dermatitis. J Dermatol Treat 2021;32(7):721–9.

Adjunctive Management of Itch in Atopic Dermatitis

Sarah G. Brooks, BA, Gil Yosipovitch, MD*

KEYWORDS

- Atopic dermatitis • Itch • Adjunctive treatment • Topical adjuncts

KEY POINTS

- Itch is the most common and burdensome symptom associated with atopic dermatitis (AD).
- Treatment of AD-associated itch can be challenging, and there is a need for adjunctive management of symptoms to improve quality of life.
- Emerging therapeutic agents may decrease the need for the use of treatments with undesirable side effects, such as topical corticosteroids.

INTRODUCTION

Atopic dermatitis (AD), also known as atopic eczema, is a chronic relapsing inflammatory skin condition that initially takes its toll on children, being seen in 15% to 30% of the pediatric population globally, with a substantial percentage persisting into adulthood.[1,2] The 1-year prevalence of diagnosed AD in adults during the last 2 decades is estimated to be between 1% and 17%.[3] AD flares can present with a wide range of clinical symptoms, most commonly dry skin that is red, itchy, or painful.[4] The most common and burdensome symptom is itching, with 85% to 92% endorsing this daily.[5,6] Itch has a substantial negative impact on quality of life due to its contribution to impaired sleep, reduced social functioning, impaired mental health, and reduced general vitality in AD patients compared to the general population.[7] Due to the complex etiology of AD, treatment can be challenging. There is often a need for adjunctive management of symptoms to reduce burden. The optimal approach must be broad and target multiple points along the itch pathway in addition to addressing external factors.[8] This article will summarize the current literature on the latest therapies used adjunctively to conventional treatment regimens.

CURRENT GUIDELINES

The foundation of baseline management for most people with AD is the use of emollients or moisturizers to minimize dryness. This method should be done in conjunction with topical corticosteroids (TCS) or topical calcineurin inhibitors such as tacrolimus or pimecrolimus, which work against pruritus by inhibiting T-lymphocyte activation and suppressing the synthesis of pro-inflammatory cytokines.[9] TCS improve itch in patients with AD rapidly, often within 1 to 4 days.[10] However, this is not a viable long-term treatment due to adverse effects.

Crisaborole ointment, a phosphodiesterase inhibitor, and ruxolitinib cream, a Janus kinase (JAK) inhibitor, are also optimized topical therapies for itch in AD.[11]

For those with more severe or widespread disease, oral agents may be required. The first-line systemic agents for AD are biologics.[11] The 2017 Food and Drug Administration (FDA) approval of dupilumab, an injectable monoclonal antibody that inhibits IL-4 and IL-13 signal transduction, has revolutionized the management of AD in individuals 6 months of age and older. The second biologic approved for the treatment of AD is subcutaneous tralokinumab, which targets IL-13 and is

Dr. Phillip Frost Department of Dermatology and Cutaneous Surgery, Miami Itch Center, University of Miami Miller School of Medicine, 5555 Ponce de Leon Boulevard, Coral Gables, FL 33146, USA
* Corresponding author. 5555 Ponce de Leon Boulevard, Coral Gables, FL 33146.
E-mail address: yosipog@gmail.com

Dermatol Clin 42 (2024) 577–589
https://doi.org/10.1016/j.det.2024.04.008
0733-8635/24/© 2024 Elsevier Inc. All rights reserved.

approved for patients over the age of 12.[12] According to the most recently updated guidelines for the management of AD, JAK inhibitors are advised for those who fail other systemic therapies.[11] The FDA-approved JAK inhibitors for AD include upadacitinib and abrocitinib, both of which preferentially target JAK-1.[11] A comprehensive treatment algorithm for AD is proposed as depicted in **Fig. 1**.

TOPICAL ADJUNCTS

Damage to the skin barrier facilitates the entry of external pathogens and irritants, triggering inflammation and itch.[13] Utilizing moisturizers may lubricate the skin (emollients), prevent water evaporation (occlusives), and retain water (humectant), counteracting increased transepidermal water loss noted in atopic itchy skin.[14] In addition to the typical ingredients found in moisturizers, several supplemental topical agents work especially well for itch in AD. A summary of topical adjunctive therapies is shown in **Table 1**.

Colloidal Oatmeal

The use of 1% colloidal oatmeal cream has been used to treat pruritic dermatoses for centuries and has demonstrated benefit as an adjunctive treatment for itch in AD.[15,16] Oatmeal contains different types of phenols as well as starches and β-D-glucans that help to create an occlusive barrier with anti-itch activity.[17,18] One study found a significant improvement in itching of AD patient at weeks 2, 4, and 8 when oatmeal cream and body wash were added to their normal topical regimen.[19] Colloidal oatmeal cream also appears to be effective in reducing itch when used instead of a patient's usual AD topical regimen.[20]

Ceramides

Ceramides normally make up 50% of the lipid bilayer within the stratum corneum; however, they are significantly reduced in atopic skin.[21] Thus, topical supplementation of ceramides is an implicated therapy for restoring barrier function and relieving certain AD symptoms, specifically itch.[22] Importantly, ceramide reduction is particularly prominent in black skin compared to white and Asian skin.[23] Given that newborns and infants are highly susceptible to skin barrier disruption, and the prevalence of AD in black children has disproportionately increased over the past 2 decades, addressing ceramide imbalance is also an important part of ameliorating racial disparities in childhood eczema.[24,25] One cohort study showed improvement of itch from "very itchy" to itching only when the skin was wet after a twice-daily regimen of ceramide-containing cleanser and moisturizer were used for 6 weeks.[26] Notably, ceramide may be used in combination with other ingredients, such as 1% pramoxine and 1% hydrocortisone, to additively ameliorate itch.[27] There is growing evidence to suggest that ceramides are a safe and effective adjunct for treating AD-associated itch and may be a suitable alternative to avoid or limit steroid-containing substances.[28–30]

Bacteria-Derived Compounds

The skin microbiome is a key player in the regulation of itch via its release of neurochemicals and communication with the skin, brain, and peripheral sensory neurons.[31,32] In AD flares, there is an overall decrease in microbial diversity and a proliferation of certain bacteria, namely *Staphylococcus aureus*

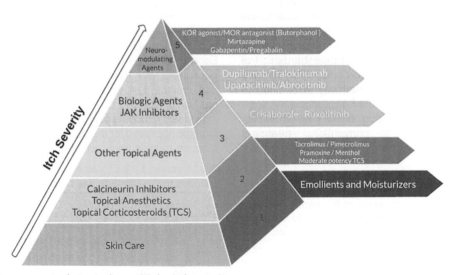

Fig. 1. Management of atopic dermatitis by itch severity.

Table 1
Atopic adjuncts for the management of atopic

Agent	Mechanism	Dose	Notes
Colloidal oatmeal	• Phenols, starches, and β-glucans create and a barrier with anti-itch activity	• 1% Cream or body wash	• Safe and gentle option for young patients
Ceramides	• Replacement of ceramide loss in lipid bilayer of stratum corneum • Restore barrier function	• 0.5%–4%	• May be used in combination with pramoxine and hydrocortisone
Bleach baths	• Restores the skin surface microbiome by eradicating bacteria, especially by decreasing the abundance of *S. aureus*	• Dilute 6% bleach to a concentration of 0.005%	• Does not worsen antibiotic resistance or disrupt epidermal barrier function
Prebiotic/probiotic (synbiotic) baths	• Alters the skin microbiome and decreases skin pH, thus reducing colonization with *S. aureus* that is driven by the increased pH in atopic skin	• Variable	• Lactic acid in particular has shown anti-pruritic effect
Topical anesthetics	• Pramoxine- interferes with impulse transmission along sensory nerve fibers • Lidocaine- inhibits voltage-gated sodium channels, reducing the firing of pruriceptive sensory fibers	• Pramoxine: 1% cream • Lidocaine: 3%–5% cream	• Pramoxine is often combined with ceramide cream for rapid and long-lasting itch relief
Cooling agents	• Menthol- unclear; potential activation of TRPM8 on C-fibers, stimulation of Aδ fibers, or activation of K-opioid receptors • Camphor- TRP activation	• Menthol: 0.5%-3% cream/ointment • Camphor: 0.5%-9% cream/ointment	• Avoid in patients who report worsening of their itch with cold showers • Menthol may irritate the skin when used in higher concentrations • Menthol and camphor are often compounded together
Mu-opioid receptor (MOR) antagonists	• Blocks the pro-pruritic effect of mu-opioid receptors	• Naltrexone 1% cream	• Further research is needed to evaluate topical vs systemic opiates to treat AD adjunctively • Opiates administered via nasal spray (butorphanol) and orally (difelikefalin) may have greater clinical utility
Cannabinoids	• N-palmitoylethanolamide (PEA)- inhibits endocannabinoid breakdown and reduce mast cell degranulation • Cannabidiol (CBD)- suppresses level of pro-inflammatory cytokines, antimicrobial properties	• 0.3% PEA cream	• CBD products containing <0.3% tetrahydrocannabinol (THC) are legal on the federal level, but it is important to check with state laws before prescribing

(*continued on next page*)

Table 1
(continued)

Agent	Mechanism	Dose	Notes
Aryl hydrocarbon receptor (AhR) agonists	• Tapinarof- binds directly to the AhR receptor, resulting in suppression of inflammatory cytokines	• 1% Tapinar of cream	• May substitute for coal tar, which can be malodorous and irritating • Promising pruritus reduction from phase III trials (ADORING 1/2) • Long-term safety anticipated by ADORING 3
Phosphodiesterase type 4 (PDE4) inhibitors	• Roflumilast- blocks PDE4 and leads to the accumulation of cyclic adenosine monophosphate (cAMP), resulting in decreased production of proinflammatory mediators/increased production of anti-inflammatory mediators	• 0.15% Roflumilast Cream	• Itch reduction may be seen as early as 24 h following application according to recent phase III trial results (INTEGUMENT 1/2)

(*S aureus*).[33] The non-histaminergic itch pathway in AD can be activated by proteases released following bacteria binding to protease-activated receptors (PAR-2 and PAR-4), which are overexpressed in the itchy skin of AD patients.[34,35] Because of this mechanism, certain therapeutic compounds that limit the overgrowth of bacteria have shown efficacy in reducing inflammation and itch.[36] *Vitreoscilla filiformis*, for example, is a nonpathogenic bacterium found in thermal springs thought to reduce pruritus in patients with AD when applied in a compounded cream by preventing biofilm formation of *S aureus*.[4,37,38] Other bacterial substances that have improved itch in AD patients include derivatives of *Pantoea agglomerans* and *Vitis vinifera* seed extract.[39,40]

Acidification of the Skin

The colonization of *S aureus* at the skin surface in eczema is largely driven by the associated increase in skin pH, often to greater than 6.5, which leads to the activation of PAR-2 receptors and induces itch.[41,42] Therefore, the acidification of skin with low-pH washes and moisturizers, such as lactic acid, can reverse the pH abnormality and reduce itch.[43–46] One recent study evaluated the efficacy of daily symbiotic baths containing 6 viable lactic acid bacteria and prebiotics in 7 patients with AD.[47] On day 9 and day 14, patients reported significantly reduced pruritus compared to placebo.[47] These results, among others, suggest that lactic acid may be an effective adjuvant topical for pruritus in eczema.[48]

Bleach Baths

Bleach baths (dilute solutions of sodium hypochlorite) have been used for a few decades as an antiseptic therapy for AD.[49,50] More recently, they have further been investigated as an inexpensive adjunctive therapy for patients with AD given their anti-inflammatory and anti-itching effects.[51,52] Infection with *S aureus* is the most frequent complication of AD, and bleach baths are useful in decreasing the abundance of *S aureus* without worsening antibiotic resistance or disrupting epidermal barrier function.[50] A randomized trial investigating the effect of twice-weekly bleach baths in adults with AD demonstrated decreased itch in 80% of subjects after 6 weeks of treatment and 100% of subjects after 12 weeks. Furthermore, 87% of subjects reported improvement in their sleep as subscore of pruritus.[53] Several other studies have reported a varied improvement in AD severity with bleach baths, although additional large clinical trials are needed.[54,55] Current guidelines support the adjunctive use of bleach baths for patients with moderate-to-severe AD, although clinical improvement may only be seen in about one-fifth of patients.[54,56] 10% of patients can be expected to have greater than 50% improvement.[54] Bleach baths are not recommended for mild cases of AD.[56]

PHOTOTHERAPY

Phototherapy for the treatment of pruritus in AD has been well-studied and is concluded to be effective, safe, and tolerable.[57] Narrowband UVB (NB-UVB) has largely replaced broadband UVB in the clinical setting given its low side effect profile and non-inferiority in pruritus reduction.[58,59] Furthermore, NB-UVB appears to reduce pruritus to a greater extent than UVA in patients with chronic AD.[60] Home phototherapy devices are also available and have demonstrated similar efficacy to office-based phototherapy with the added benefit of cost reduction and increased patient adherence.[61] Evidence demonstrating the impact of different types of phototherapy on itch has thus far been largely variable and of low certainty, emphasizing the need for further research in this area.[62]

TOPICAL NEUROMODULATORS

There is a growing body of evidence to suggest that the nervous system plays a substantial role in promoting AD and mediating itch.[63] The use of systemic neuromodulators or topical anesthetics, when used consistently, may be a viable way to dampen itch signaling.[8]

Anesthetics

Topical anesthetics, such as lidocaine, polidocanol, and pramoxine, have shown some efficacy in AD given their anti-inflammatory and anti-pruritic properties.[64] Pramoxine may reduce itch duration and magnitude by interfering with impulse transmission along sensory nerve fibers.
[65,66] Furthermore, pramoxine may be used in combination with other compounds to provide both moisturization and antipruritic effects.[67] Patients with AD who have used daily ceramide cream with 1% pramoxine hydrochloride found it to provide both rapid and long-lasting relief of itch.[27] A striking 87.5% reported relief of nighttime itch.[27] Lidocaine alleviates itch in AD by inhibiting voltage-gated sodium channels, thus reducing the firing of nociceptive and pruriceptive sensory fibers.[8,64] Additionally, a topical preparation containing 3% polidocanol, an anesthetic surfactant, and 5% urea led to a significant reduction in itch associated with various pruritic skin conditions, including AD, in a multicenter trial.[68] The use of topical anesthetics as an adjunctive treatment in AD requires further large-group studies to assess efficacy.

Cooling Agents

The use of cooling agents as adjunctive treatment may modulate the perception of itch in AD by evoking the sensation of cold. Common cooling agents include menthol, camphor, and phenol.[8]

The exact antipruritic mechanism of menthol is not entirely clear, but some postulate the activation of TRPM8 on C-fibers, direct stimulation of A-delta fibers, or activation of kappa-opioid receptors.[69,70] One study assessed the application of 3% menthol-containing cream in 18 patients with AD and reported a significant reduction in itch at 1 month.[71] In another study of 35 children, 7 days of using a sprayable menthol product led to improved itch.[72] Menthol combined with ceramide and polidocanol has also shown efficacy in reducing itch in AD patients within as little as 5 minutes after application.[73] Camphor similarly functions through TRP activation; however, it potentiates both heat and cold sensations and functions at the TRP vanilloid-3 (TRPV3) and TRPM8 ion channels.[74,75] Of note these topicals should not be administered to a subset of patients with atopic eczema, (approximately 30%), who report that cold temperatures or cold showers aggravate their itch.[76] Additional studies are needed to evaluate the efficacy of these agents in AD, especially menthol, as it may act as an irritant to the skin when used in higher concentrations.[77–79]

Cannabinoids

Cannabinoid receptors 1 and 2 (CB1 and CB2) are abundant in cutaneous nerve fibers, mast cells, and keratinocytes.[77] The use of topical compounds containing N-palmitoylethanolamine (PEA), an endocannabinoid-like lipid mediator, has shown relief of pruritus in patients with chronic itch conditions, including AD, likely due in part to the inhibition of endocannabinoid breakdown and the reduction of mast cell degranulation.[78,79] In a large multicentric, prospective, cohort study, patients reported an improved quality of life secondary to reduced pruritus and improved sleep quality with PEA 0.3% cream.[78] Of note, this study also reported that 56% of patients no longer needed to use topical corticosteroids with the addition of PEA, suggesting that this could be a beneficial adjunctive treatment for AD in place of regimens with harsh side effect profiles. One study evaluated topical adelmidrol, an analog of PEA, in a group of 20 pediatric patients with mild AD. Complete lesion clearance was noted in 80% of patients with no side effects, providing some evidence for the safety of these agents in children.[80] However, this was a singular pilot study and additional controlled clinical trials are needed. Phytocannabinoids, such as cannabidiol, are increasingly being studied for their anti-inflammatory effects, and have similarly shown efficacy in reducing the intensity of AD-associated pruritus and other symptoms.[81,82]

Coal Tar and Aryl Hydrocarbon Receptor Agonists

Coal tar has a long history of use in patients with psoriasis and AD for itch reduction, although its use is declining, and its efficacy is only moderate.[83,84] Coal tar activates the aryl hydrocarbon receptors (AhR) in keratinocytes, resulting in the induction of epidermal differentiation, restoration of major skin barrier proteins including filaggrin, and subsequent downregulation of the inflammatory process in the skin.[85] AhR is thus a promising key target for pharmacologic effects.[86]

ANTIHISTAMINES

To date, there is no concrete proof that oral nonsedating antihistamines, such as cetirizine, reduce pruritus in atopic dermatitis, and therefore they are not recommended.[87] The intermittent use of sedating antihistamines such as diphenhydramine and hydroxyzine may be useful for helping patients sleep through the night without waking to scratch.[88] Doxepin is a tricyclic antidepressant that is a potent H1 and H2 antagonist and has been used as adjunctive management in AD. One randomized controlled trial conducted in 270 patients reported relief of pruritus in 85% of patients treated with 5% doxepin cream compared to 57% of the vehicle-treated patients.[89] Nonetheless, its use is limited by sedation from percutaneous absorption and high rates of contact dermatitis.[90] Both topical and oral antihistamines may cause anticholinergic symptoms including dry mouth, blurred vision, and tachycardia.[91] Furthermore, their use may lead to reduced sleep quality and decreased rapid eye movement sleep, which is especially important to consider in children.[88] Given the substantial adverse effects and limited efficacy, antihistamines should be considered lower on the list of adjunctive treatments for AD.

SYSTEMIC NEUROMODULATORS

Serotonin receptors are widely distributed in the skin, including in peripheral sensory nerves, keratinocytes, and mast cells, lending to their reported antipruritic effect in various dermatologic conditions.[92,93] Fluvoxamine and paroxetine are 2 selective serotonin reuptake inhibitors that have demonstrated efficacy in patients with pruritus of varying etiologies.[92] Mirtazapine is a dual-acting antidepressant that blocks both serotonergic and noradrenergic receptors and has additional H1-antihistamine properties.[94] Furthermore, its sedating properties may play a role in nocturnal itch reduction and subsequent improved sleep

quality, supporting its use in AD patients with symptom exacerbation during sleep.[95,96]

Antiepileptics such as gabapentin and pregabalin have gained substantial attention in the dermatologic community for treating neuropathic itch. Although AD is not neuropathic in origin, there is significant involvement of neural dysregulation and hypersensitization.[34] Gabapentin and pregabalin act on voltage-gated calcium channels, which subsequently regulate the release of substance P (SP) and calcitonin gene-related peptide (CGRP) and reduce neural sensitization.[97] Studies have found an elevated density of SP-positive dermal nerve fibers and elevated cutaneous levels of SP in patients with itch secondary to AD.[98,99] These findings provide support for the potential role of antiepileptics in treating atopic pruritus.

OPIATES

Mu-opioid receptor (MOR) agonism has a pro-pruritic effect, while kappa-opioid receptor (KOR) agonism has an anti-pruritic effect.[100] Therefore MOR antagonists and KOR agonists may provide therapeutic benefits in reducing pruritus in AD.

Mu-opioid Receptor Modulators

In a series of 2 studies, the efficacy of naltrexone, a MOR antagonist, was tested. In the initial pilot study of 18 patients with varying pruritic conditions including AD, more than 70% of patients experienced significant itch relief after treatment with 1% naltrexone cream.[101] In a subsequent cross-over trial of 40 patients with AD, the researchers found that the cream containing naltrexone was 29.4% more effective in reducing pruritus and worked about 30 minutes faster compared to the placebo.[101] Prior studies have shown comparable results, providing some evidence for the role of peripheral opioid receptors in atopic itch.[102,103] Further research is needed to evaluate whether topical or oral agents would be the most effective adjuncts for treating AD.

Kappa-opioid Receptor Modulators

Dysregulation in the κ-opioid system is thought to contribute to chronic itch by acting on both the peripheral and central nervous systems.[104] We previously reported that butorphanol, a KOR agonist and MOR antagonist, has antipruritic effects in different types of chronic itch including severe AD.[105,106] In a recent phase II clinical trial, 3 oral doses of KOR agonist difelikefalin were evaluated for their impact on pruritus intensity in patients with moderate to severe AD, all of which reduced itch compared to placebo.[107] However, a recent phase III trial did not achieve a significant antipruritic effect. Another KOR agonist of interest includes oral asimadoline, which significantly reduced nighttime itching in a multi-site proof-of-concept RCT of 221 subjects with AD; however, it similarly did not achieve the primary endpoint efficacy in a phase III trial.[108]

COMPLEMENTARY AND ALTERNATIVE THERAPIES
Targeting Stress

In addition to targeting the internal pathways associated with AD, it is important to also address external stressors that may trigger worsening disease. While new drugs may be able to adequately manage symptoms, psychologic stress can lead to a vicious cycle of scratching, provoking the relapse of AD symptoms regardless of any positive drug effect.[109,110] Studies have found that relief of cervical muscle tension and massage therapy may be useful adjunctive therapies.[111,112] In one study assessing the efficacy of massage therapy in young children with AD in addition to their existing topical regimen, 1 month of daily, 20-min sessions led to significant improvement of redness, scaling, lichenification, and pruritus, as well as decreased anxiety levels in both the children and their parents.[112]

Acupuncture

Acupuncture is an alternative therapy involving the insertion of thin needles into the skin.[8] In a recent trial assessing the impact of acupuncture on symptoms of AD, 30 participants underwent 4 weeks of acupuncture and reported significant improvement in itch severity.[113] Despite proof that acupuncture is effective in the management of AD, its mechanism is not entirely known. There is some evidence to show that acupuncture may ameliorate skin inflammation and serotonergic itch through the blockade of serotonin 5-HT2 and 5-HT7 receptors.[114] The antipruritic effects of acupuncture may involve vasodilation or stimulation of inflammatory cell mediators, depletion of neurotransmitters through the activation of C fibers, and reduction of type I hypersensitivity reactions.[115,116]

Dietary Supplements

Omega-3 (n-3) and omega-6 (n-6) are essential fatty acids (FAs) that contribute to the formation of ceramides and thus are important in the maintenance of the optimal skin barrier.[117] The typical western diet tends to favor excess n-6 FAs, potentially resulting in a shortage of n-3 FAs. Given that n-3 FAs are associated with decreased inflammation, this imbalance may lead to the itch associated with AD.[118] Thus, targeting an ideal n-3:n-6 FA ratio through the consumption of healthy food is advised as a feasible, low-risk supplemental regimen.[119] Evening primrose oil and borage oil are other n-6 compounds that are rich in gamma-linolenic acid. When applied topically, these oils can reduce eczema severity and itch.[120,121]

EMERGING TOPICAL THERAPIES
Phosphodiesterase Type 4 Inhibitors

Crisaborole ointment is a phosphodiesterase type 4 (PDE4) inhibitor that is approved for the treatment of mild-to-moderate AD in patients as young as 3 months of age. Given its efficacy and safety as a nonsteroidal topical agent, additional PDE4 inhibitors are under development and entering the market. Roflumilast cream, for instance, is approved for the treatment of plaque psoriasis and recently showed favorable results in a phase III trial for AD. Inhibiting PDE4 has anti-inflammatory as well as an early and distinct antipruritic effect.[122,123] In children aged 2 to 5, roflumilast 0.05% cream provided a quick reduction of itch, with 35.3% of patients achieving a 4-point reduction on the Worst-Itch Numeric Rating Scale at week 4.[124] Recent data from 2 phase III trials (INTEGUMENT-1 and INTEGUMENT-2) demonstrated a rapid and significant reduction in itch in adults and children over the age of 6 with mild to moderate AD following application of roflumilast cream 0.15%.[125] Benefits were seen in as little as 24 hours following the initial application. The cream was well tolerated and had minimal adverse events that were limited to 3.5% of subjects.[125]

Aryl Hydrocarbon Receptor Agonists

Tapinarof is an AhR agonist that has demonstrated significant improvement of pruritus in AD.[126] A phase II trial found that the reduction in pruritus from baseline to each study visit up to week 8 was greater in AD patients treated with tapinarof 1% cream than those treated with vehicle, with a clear separation between the 2 groups emerging at week 2.[127] To date, 2 out of 3 subsequent phase III trials (ADORING 2 and ADORING 1) have reported promising results that are consistent with phase II data. The use of tapinarof 1% cream daily in adults and children as young as 2 years old had a meaningful impact on itch reduction in 52.8% and 55.8% of subjects at week 8, respectively.[128,129] The highly anticipated final trial (ADORING 3) will provide insight into the long-term safety of tapinarof for patients with AD.

SUMMARY AND FUTURE DIRECTIONS

Itch is by far the most common complaint of AD patients. Despite the efficacy of first-line therapies and the ongoing development of new targeted drugs, the itch can still be difficult to control. Furthermore, several widely used therapies such as TCS and immunosuppressants are accompanied by adverse effects that patients would prefer to avoid. Navigating this condition requires therapies to control vicious itch-scratch cycles and minimize the burden on quality of life. The adjunctive management of itch AD is thus an important and comprehensive option that should be offered to all patients when creating a personalized therapeutic approach. The data presented in this review highlight the most up-to-date adjunctive agents with supporting evidence for itch-reduction.

CLINICS CARE POINTS

- Patients with AD should be asked about the severity of their itch and the impact it may be having on their daily activities.
- Patients should be offered adjunctive therapy if itch is not adequately controlled with common agents.
- Clinicians should be prepared to discuss the benefits and risks of adjunctive management when creating a personalized treatment approach.

DISCLOSURE

Dr G. Yosipovitch has received funding or grants from Sanofi, France, Regeneron Pharmaceuticals, United States, Pfizer, United States, Escient Health, Novartis, Switzerland, Eli Lilly, Celldex, United States, and Kiniksa Pharmaceuticals, United States. He has participated on a Data Safety Monitoring/Advisory board and received consulting support from Abbive, Arcutis, Escient Health, Eli Lilly, Galderma, LEO Pharma, Novartis, Pfizer, Pierre Fabre, Regeneron Pharmaceuticals Inc., Sanofi, Trevi Therapeutics, Vifor, Kamari, Kiniksa, and GSK. Patents include Topical Acetaminophen Formulations for Itch Relief.

REFERENCES

1. Silverberg JI. Public health burden and epidemiology of atopic dermatitis. Dermatol Clin 2017; 35(3):283–9.

2. Raimondo A, Lembo S. Atopic dermatitis: epidemiology and clinical phenotypes. Dermatol Pract Concept 2021;11(4):e2021146.

3. Bylund S, von Kobyletzki LB, Svalstedt M, et al. Prevalence and incidence of atopic dermatitis: a systematic review. Acta Derm Venereol 2020; 100(12):320–9.

4. Patsatsi A, Vakirlis E, Kanelleas A, et al. Effect of a novel "emollient plus" formulation on mild-to-severe atopic dermatitis and other dry skin-related diseases as monotherapy or adjunctive therapy: an observational study on efficacy, tolerance and quality of life in adult patients. Eur J Dermatol 2023;33(2):137–46.

5. Dawn A, Papoiu AD, Chan YH, et al. Itch characteristics in atopic dermatitis: results of a web-based questionnaire. Br J Dermatol 2009;160(3):642–4.

6. Simpson EL, Bieber T, Eckert L, et al. Patient burden of moderate to severe atopic dermatitis (AD): Insights from a phase 2b clinical trial of dupilumab in adults. J Am Acad Dermatol 2016;74(3):491–8.

7. Kiebert G, Sorensen SV, Revicki D, et al. Atopic dermatitis is associated with a decrement in health-related quality of life. Int J Dermatol 2002; 41(3):151–8.

8. Elmariah SB. Adjunctive management of itch in atopic dermatitis. Dermatol Clin 2017;35(3):373–94.

9. Gutfreund K, Bienias W, Szewczyk A, et al. Topical calcineurin inhibitors in dermatology. Part I: Properties, method and effectiveness of drug use. Postepy Dermatol Alergol 2013;30(3):165–9.

10. Wahlgren C-F, Hägermark Ö, Bergström R, et al. Evaluation of a new method of assessing pruritus and antipruritic drugs. Skin Pharmacol 2009;1(1): 3–13.

11. Davis DMR, Drucker AM, Alikhan A, et al. Guidelines of care for the management of atopic dermatitis in adults with phototherapy and systemic therapies. J Am Acad Dermatol 2023;90(2): e43–56.

12. Pezzolo E, Sechi A, Tartaglia J, et al. A critical evaluation of suitability of tralokinumab for treatment of moderate-to-severe atopic dermatitis in adolescents and adults. Expert Rev Clin Immunol 2023; 20(3):255–66.

13. Elmariah SB, Lerner EA. Topical therapies for pruritus. Semin Cutan Med Surg 2011;30(2):118–26.

14. Breternitz M, Kowatzki D, Langenauer M, et al. Placebo-controlled, double-blind, randomized, prospective study of a glycerol-based emollient on eczematous skin in atopic dermatitis: biophysical and clinical evaluation. Skin Pharmacol Physiol 2008;21(1):39–45.

15. Diluvio L, Dattola A, Cannizzaro MV, et al. Clinical and confocal evaluation of avenanthramides-based daily cleansing and emollient cream in pediatric population affected by atopic dermatitis and

xerosis. G Ital Dermatol Venereol 2019;154(1): 32–6.

16. Reynertson KA, Garay M, Nebus J, et al. Anti-inflammatory activities of colloidal oatmeal (Avena sativa) contribute to the effectiveness of oats in treatment of itch associated with dry, irritated skin. J Drugs Dermatol 2015;14(1):43–8.

17. Fowler JF, Nebus J, Wallo W, et al. Colloidal oatmeal formulations as adjunct treatments in atopic dermatitis. J Drugs Dermatol 2012;11(7): 804–7.

18. Sur R, Nigam A, Grote D, et al. Avenanthramides, polyphenols from oats, exhibit anti-inflammatory and anti-itch activity. Arch Dermatol Res 2008; 300(10):569–74.

19. Nebus J, Nystrand G, Fowler J, et al. A daily oat-based skin care regimen for atopic skin. J Am Acad Derm 2009;60(3 Supplement 1):AB67.

20. Therapeutic benefits of an over-the-counter daily moisturizing 1% colloidal oatmeal cream on dry, itchy skin due to atopic dermatitis. J Am Acad Dermatol 2015;72(5, Supplement 1):AB76.

21. Harrison IP, Spada F. Breaking the itch-scratch cycle: topical options for the management of chronic cutaneous itch in atopic dermatitis. Medicines (Basel) 2019;6(3):76.

22. Nugroho WT, Sawitri S, Astindari A, et al. The efficacy of moisturisers containing ceramide compared with other moisturisers in the management of atopic dermatitis: a systematic literature review and meta-analysis. Indian J Dermatol 2023;68(1):53–8.

23. Gan C, Mahil S, Pink A, et al. Atopic dermatitis in skin of colour. Part 1: new discoveries in epidemiology and pathogenesis. Clin Exp Dermatol 2023; 48(6):609–16.

24. Schachner LA, Andriessen A, Benjamin L, et al. Racial and ethnic variations in skin barrier properties and cultural practices in skin of color newborns, infants, and children. J Drugs Dermatol 2023;22(7):657–63.

25. Choragudi S, Yosipovitch G. Trends in the prevalence of eczema among US children by age, sex, race, and ethnicity from 1997 to 2018. JAMA Dermatology 2023;159(4):454–6.

26. Lynde CW, Andriessen A. A cohort study on a ceramide-containing cleanser and moisturizer used for atopic dermatitis. Cutis 2014;93(4):207–13.

27. Zirwas MJ, Barkovic S. Anti-pruritic efficacy of itch relief lotion and cream in patients with atopic history: comparison with hydrocortisone cream. J Drugs Dermatol 2017;16(3):243–7.

28. Draelos ZD, Raymond I. The efficacy of a ceramide-based cream in mild-to-moderate atopic dermatitis. J Clin Aesthet Dermatol 2018;11(5): 30–2.

29. Spada F, Harrison IP, Barnes TM, et al. A daily regimen of a ceramide-dominant moisturizing cream and cleanser restores the skin permeability barrier in adults with moderate eczema: A randomized trial. Dermatol Ther 2021;34(4):e14970.

30. Yang Q, Liu M, Li X, et al. The benefit of a ceramide-linoleic acid-containing moisturizer as an adjunctive therapy for a set of xerotic dermatoses. Dermatol Ther 2019;32(4):e13017.

31. Li W, Yosipovitch G. The Role of the microbiome and microbiome-derived metabolites in atopic dermatitis and non-histaminergic itch. Am J Clin Dermatol 2020;21(Suppl 1):44–50.

32. Kim HS, Yosipovitch G. The skin microbiota and itch: is there a link? J Clin Med 2020;9(4):1190.

33. Kong HH, Oh J, Deming C, et al. Temporal shifts in the skin microbiome associated with disease flares and treatment in children with atopic dermatitis. Genome Res 2012;22(5):850–9.

34. Yosipovitch G, Rosen JD, Hashimoto T. Itch: From mechanism to (novel) therapeutic approaches. J Allergy Clin Immunol 2018;142(5):1375–90.

35. Nattkemper LA, Tey HL, Valdes-Rodriguez R, et al. The genetics of chronic itch: gene expression in the skin of patients with atopic dermatitis and psoriasis with severe itch. J Invest Dermatol 2018; 138(6):1311–7.

36. Zeichner J, Seite S. From probiotic to prebiotic using thermal spring water. J Drugs Dermatol 2018; 17(6):657–62.

37. Park HY, Kim CR, Huh IS, et al. Staphylococcus aureus colonization in acute and chronic skin lesions of patients with atopic dermatitis. Ann Dermatol 2013;25(4):410–6.

38. Gueniche A, Knaudt B, Schuck E, et al. Effects of nonpathogenic gram-negative bacterium Vitreoscilla filiformis lysate on atopic dermatitis: a prospective, randomized, double-blind, placebo-controlled clinical study. Br J Dermatol 2008;159(6):1357–63.

39. Nakai K, Kubota Y, Soma GI, et al. The effect of lipopolysaccharide-containing moisturizing cream on skin care in patients with mild atopic dermatitis. In Vivo 2019;33(1):109–14.

40. Belloni G, Pinelli S, Veraldi S. A randomised, double-blind, vehicle-controlled study to evaluate the efficacy and safety of MAS063D (Atopiclair) in the treatment of mild to moderate atopic dermatitis. Eur J Dermatol 2005;15(1):31–6.

41. Ali SM, Yosipovitch G. Skin pH: from basic science to basic skin care. Acta Derm Venereol 2013;93(3): 261–7.

42. Jang H, Matsuda A, Jung K, et al. Skin pH is the master switch of kallikrein 5-mediated skin barrier destruction in a murine atopic dermatitis model. J Invest Dermatol 2016;136(1):127–35.

43. Simon D, Nobbe S, Nägeli M, et al. Short- and long-term effects of two emollients on itching and skin restoration in xerotic eczema. Dermatol Ther 2018;31(6):e12692.

44. Jaeger T, Rothmaier M, Zander H, et al. Acid-coated textiles (pH 5.5-6.5)–a new therapeutic strategy for atopic eczema? Acta Derm Venereol 2015;95(6):659–63.

45. Panther DJ, Jacob SE. The importance of acidification in atopic eczema: an underexplored avenue for treatment. J Clin Med 2015;4(5):970–8.

46. Lee NR, Lee HJ, Yoon NY, et al. Acidic water bathing could be a safe and effective therapeutic modality for severe and refractory atopic dermatitis. Ann Dermatol 2016;28(1):126–9.

47. Noll M, Jäger M, Lux L, et al. Improvement of atopic dermatitis by synbiotic baths. Microorganisms 2021;9(3):527.

48. Niccoli AA, Artesi AL, Candio F, et al. Preliminary results on clinical effects of probiotic lactobacillus salivarius LS01 in children affected by atopic dermatitis. J Clin Gastroenterol 2014;48.

49. Huang SM, Chen YY, Chen YC, et al. 0.005 % hypochlorite reduces serine protease in cultured human keratinocytes: Evidences supporting bleach bath improves atopic dermatitis. J Dermatol Sci 2022;107(3):169–72.

50. Huang JT, Abrams M, Tlougan B, et al. Treatment of Staphylococcus aureus colonization in atopic dermatitis decreases disease severity. Pediatrics 2009;123(5):e808–14.

51. Paller AS, Beck LA. Bleach baths for atopic dermatitis: Evidence of efficacy but more data are needed. Ann Allergy Asthma Immunol 2022; 128(6):617–8.

52. Krynicka K, Trzeciak M. The role of sodium hypochlorite in atopic dermatitis therapy: a narrative review. Int J Dermatol 2022;61(9):1080–6.

53. Stolarczyk A, Perez-Nazario N, Knowlden SA, et al. Bleach baths enhance skin barrier, reduce itch but do not normalize skin dysbiosis in atopic dermatitis. Arch Dermatol Res 2023;315(10):2883–92.

54. Bakaa L, Pernica JM, Couban RJ, et al. Bleach baths for atopic dermatitis: A systematic review and meta-analysis including unpublished data, Bayesian interpretation, and GRADE. Ann Allergy Asthma Immunol 2022;128(6):660–8.e669.

55. Wong SM, Ng TG, Baba R. Efficacy and safety of sodium hypochlorite (bleach) baths in patients with moderate to severe atopic dermatitis in Malaysia. J Dermatol 2013;40(11):874–80.

56. Chu DK, Schneider L, Asiniwasis RN, et al. Atopic dermatitis (eczema) guidelines: 2023 American Academy of Allergy, Asthma and Immunology/ American College of Allergy, Asthma and Immunology Joint Task Force on Practice Parameters GRADE- and Institute of Medicine-based recommendations. Ann Allergy Asthma Immunol 2024; 132(3):274–312.

57. Rivard J, Lim HW. Ultraviolet phototherapy for pruritus. Dermatol Ther 2005;18(4):344–54.

58. Kupsa R, Gruber-Wackernagel A, Hofer A, et al. Narrowband-ultraviolet B vs broadband-ultraviolet B in treatment of chronic pruritus: a randomized, single-blinded, non-inferiority study. Acta Derm Venereol 2023;103:adv9403.

59. Singer S, Berneburg M. Phototherapy. J Dtsch Dermatol Ges 2018;16(9):1120–9.

60. Legat FJ, Hofer A, Brabek E, et al. Narrowband UV-B vs medium-dose UV-A1 phototherapy in chronic atopic dermatitis. Arch Dermatol 2003; 139(2):223–4.

61. Jacob J, Pona A, Cline A, et al. Home UV phototherapy. Dermatol Clin 2020;38(1):109–26.

62. Musters AH, Mashayekhi S, Harvey J, et al. Phototherapy for atopic eczema. Cochrane Database Syst Rev 2021;10(10):Cd013870.

63. Misery L. Atopic dermatitis and the nervous system. Clin Rev Allergy Immunol 2011;41(3):259–66.

64. Sun PY, Li HG, Xu QY, et al. Lidocaine alleviates inflammation and pruritus in atopic dermatitis by blocking different population of sensory neurons. Br J Pharmacol 2023;180(10):1339–61.

65. Litt J. Topical treatments of itching without corticosteroids. Itch mechanisms and management of pruritus. New York: McGraw-Hill; 1994. p. 383.

66. Yosipovitch G, Maibach HI. Effect of topical pramoxine on experimentally induced pruritus in humans. J Am Acad Dermatol 1997;37(2 Pt 1): 278–80.

67. Agarwal A, Das A, Hassanandani T, et al. Topical pramoxine in chronic pruritus: where do we stand? Indian J Dermatol 2021;66(5):576.

68. Freitag G, Höppner T. Results of a postmarketing drug monitoring survey with a polidocanol-urea preparation for dry, itching skin. Curr Med Res Opin 1997;13(9):529–37.

69. Bromm B, Scharein E, Darsow U, et al. Effects of menthol and cold on histamine-induced itch and skin reactions in man. Neurosci Lett 1995;187(3): 157–60.

70. Galeotti N, Di Cesare Mannelli L, Mazzanti G, et al. Menthol: a natural analgesic compound. Neurosci Lett 2002;322(3):145–8.

71. Tey HL, Tay EY, Tan WD. Safety and antipruritic efficacy of a menthol-containing moisturizing cream. Skinmed 2017;15(6):437–9.

72. Riser R, Kowcz A, Schoelermann A, et al. PA-30 Tolerance profile and efficacy of a menthol-containing itch relief spray in children and atopics. Br J Dermatol Suppl 2003;149:83.

73. Umborowati MA, Nurasrifah D, Indramaya DM, et al. The role of ceramide, menthol, and polidocanol on pruritus, skin barrier function, and disease severity of mild atopic dermatitis. J Pak Assoc Dermatol 2020;30(1):98–105.

74. Sherkheli MA, Benecke H, Doerner JF, et al. Monoterpenoids induce agonist-specific desensitization

of transient receptor potential vanilloid-3 (TRPV3) ion channels. J Pharm Pharm Sci 2009;12(1): 116–28.

75. Selescu T, Ciobanu AC, Dobre C, et al. Camphor activates and sensitizes transient receptor potential melastatin 8 (TRPM8) to cooling and icilin. Chem Senses 2013;38(7):563–75.

76. Yosipovitch G, Duque MI, Fast K, et al. Scratching and noxious heat stimuli inhibit itch in humans: a psychophysical study. Br J Dermatol 2007;156(4): 629–34.

77. Ständer S, Schmelz M, Metze D, et al. Distribution of cannabinoid receptor 1 (CB1) and 2 (CB2) on sensory nerve fibers and adnexal structures in human skin. J Dermatol Sci 2005;38(3):177–88.

78. Eberlein B, Eicke C, Reinhardt HW, et al. Adjuvant treatment of atopic eczema: assessment of an emollient containing N-palmitoylethanolamine (ATOPA study). J Eur Acad Dermatol Venereol 2008;22(1): 73–82.

79. Ständer S, Reinhardt HW, Luger TA. [Topical cannabinoid agonists. An effective new possibility for treating chronic pruritus]. Hautarzt 2006;57(9): 801–7.

80. Pulvirenti N, Nasca M, Micali G. Topical adelmidrol 2% emulsion, a novel aliamide, in the treatment of mild atopic dermatitis in pediatric subjects: A pilot study. Acta Dermatovenerol Croat : ADC 2007;15: 80–3.

81. Maghfour J, Rundle CW, Rietcheck HR, et al. Assessing the effects of topical cannabidiol in patients with atopic dermatitis. Dermatol Online J 2021;27(2).

82. Maghfour J, Rietcheck HR, Rundle CW, et al. An observational study of the application of a topical cannabinoid gel on sensitive dry skin. J Drugs Dermatol 2020;19(12):1204–8.

83. Wollenberg A, Oranje A, Deleuran M, et al. ETFAD/ EADV Eczema task force 2015 position paper on diagnosis and treatment of atopic dermatitis in adult and paediatric patients. J Eur Acad Dermatol Venereol 2016;30(5):729–47.

84. Slutsky JB, Clark RA, Remedios AA, et al. An evidence-based review of the efficacy of coal tar preparations in the treatment of psoriasis and atopic dermatitis. J Drugs Dermatol 2010;9(10):1258–64.

85. Smits JPH, Ederveen THA, Rikken G, et al. Targeting the cutaneous microbiota in atopic dermatitis by coal tar via AHR-dependent induction of antimicrobial peptides. J Invest Dermatol 2020;140(2): 415–24.e410.

86. van den Bogaard EH, Bergboer JG, Vonk-Bergers M, et al. Coal tar induces AHR-dependent skin barrier repair in atopic dermatitis. J Clin Invest 2013; 123(2):917–27.

87. Frazier W, Bhardwaj N. Atopic dermatitis: diagnosis and treatment. Am Fam Physician 2020;101(10): 590–8.

88. He A, Feldman SR, Fleischer AB. An assessment of the use of antihistamines in the management of atopic dermatitis. J Am Acad Dermatol 2018;79(1): 92–6.

89. Drake LA, Fallon JD, Sober A. Relief of pruritus in patients with atopic dermatitis after treatment with topical doxepin cream. the doxepin study group. J Am Acad Dermatol 1994;31(4):613–6.

90. Shelley WB, Shelley ED, Talanin NY. Self-potentiating allergic contact dermatitis caused by doxepin hydrochloride cream. J Am Acad Dermatol 1996;34(1):143–4.

91. Greaves MW. Antihistamines in dermatology. Skin Pharmacol Physiol 2005;18(5):220–9.

92. Ständer S, Böckenholt B, Schürmeyer-Horst F, et al. Treatment of chronic pruritus with the selective serotonin re-uptake inhibitors paroxetine and fluvoxamine: results of an open-labelled, two-arm proof-of-concept study. Acta Derm Venereol 2009;89(1):45–51.

93. Patel P, Patel K, Pandher K, et al. The role of psychiatric, analgesic, and antiepileptic medications in chronic pruritus. Cureus 2021;13(8):e17260.

94. Anttila SA, Leinonen EV. A review of the pharmacological and clinical profile of mirtazapine. CNS Drug Rev 2001;7(3):249–64.

95. Khanna R, Boozalis E, Belzberg M, et al. Mirtazapine for the treatment of chronic pruritus. Medicines (Basel) 2019;6(3):73.

96. Davis MP, Frandsen JL, Walsh D, et al. Mirtazapine for pruritus. J Pain Symptom Manag 2003;25(3): 288–91.

97. Lee S. Pharmacological inhibition of voltage-gated Ca(2+) channels for chronic pain relief. Curr Neuropharmacol 2013;11(6):606–20.

98. Järvikallio A, Harvima IT, Naukkarinen A. Mast cells, nerves and neuropeptides in atopic dermatitis and nummular eczema. Arch Dermatol Res 2003;295(1):2–7.

99. Pincelli C, Fantini F, Massimi P, et al. Neuropeptides in skin from patients with atopic dermatitis: an immunohistochemical study. Br J Dermatol 1990; 122(6):745–50.

100. Ádám D, Arany J, Tóth KF, et al. Opioidergic signaling—a neglected, yet potentially important player in atopic dermatitis. Int J Mol Sci 2022; 23(8):4140.

101. Bigliardi PL, Stammer H, Jost G, et al. Treatment of pruritus with topically applied opiate receptor antagonist. J Am Acad Dermatol 2007;56(6): 979–88.

102. Brune A, Metze D, Luger TA, et al. Antipruritische Therapie mit dem oralen opiatrezeptorantagonisten Naltrexon. Hautarzt 2004;55(12):1130–6.

103. Metze D, Reimann S, Beissert S, et al. Efficacy and safety of naltrexone, an oral opiate receptor antagonist, in the treatment of pruritus in internal and

dermatological diseases. J Am Acad Dermatol 1999;41(4):533–9.

104. Kim BS, Inan S, Ständer S, et al. Role of kappa-opioid and mu-opioid receptors in pruritus: Peripheral and central itch circuits. Exp Dermatol 2022; 31(12):1900–7.

105. Labib A, Ju T, Lipman ZM, et al. Evaluating the Effectiveness of Intranasal Butorphanol in Reducing Chronic Itch. Acta Derm Venereol 2022;102: adv00729.

106. Dawn AG, Yosipovitch G. Butorphanol for treatment of intractable pruritus. J Am Acad Dermatol 2006; 54(3):527–31.

107. Guttman-Yassky E, Facheris P, Da Rosa JC, et al. Oral difelikefalin reduces moderate to severe pruritus and expression of pruritic and inflammatory biomarkers in subjects with atopic dermatitis. J Allergy Clin Immunol 2023;152(4):916–26.

108. Tioga Pharmaceuticals' asimadoline reduces nighttime itching and improves disease-related quality of life in patients with atopic dermatitis [press release]. San Diego, CA: Tioga Pharmaceuticals Inc.; 2017.

109. Hosono S, Fujita K, Nimura A, et al. Release of cervical muscle tension improves psychological stress and symptoms of moderate-to-severe atopic dermatitis: a case series with 20 patients. Dermatol Ther (Heidelb) 2022;12(10):2383–95.

110. Sanders KM, Akiyama T. The vicious cycle of itch and anxiety. Neurosci Biobehav Rev 2018;87: 17–26.

111. Bae BG, Oh SH, Park CO, et al. Progressive muscle relaxation therapy for atopic dermatitis: objective assessment of efficacy. Acta Derm Venereol 2012;92(1):57–61.

112. Schachner L, Field T, Hernandez-Reif M, et al. Atopic dermatitis symptoms decreased in children following massage therapy. Pediatr Dermatol 1998; 15(5):390–5.

113. Kang S, Kim Y-K, Yeom M, et al. Acupuncture improves symptoms in patients with mild-to-moderate atopic dermatitis: A randomized, sham-controlled preliminary trial. Compl Ther Med 2018; 41:90–8.

114. Park H-J, Ahn S, Lee H, et al. Acupuncture ameliorates not only atopic dermatitis-like skin inflammation but also acute and chronic serotonergic itch possibly through blockade of 5-HT2 and 5-HT7 receptors in mice. Brain Behav Immun 2021;93: 399–408.

115. Pfab F, Kirchner MT, Huss-Marp J, et al. Acupuncture compared with oral antihistamine for type I hypersensitivity itch and skin response in adults with atopic dermatitis: a patient- and examiner-blinded, randomized, placebo-controlled, crossover trial. Allergy 2012;67(4):566–73.

116. Carlsson CP, Wallengren J. Therapeutic and experimental therapeutic studies on acupuncture and itch: review of the literature. J Eur Acad Dermatol Venereol 2010;24(9):1013–6.

117. Elias PM, Gruber R, Crumrine D, et al. Formation and functions of the corneocyte lipid envelope (CLE). Biochim Biophys Acta 2014;1841(3):314–8.

118. Weylandt KH, Chiu C-Y, Gomolka B, et al. Omega-3 fatty acids and their lipid mediators: Towards an understanding of resolvin and protectin formation. Prostag Other Lipid Mediat 2012;97(3):73–82.

119. Labib A, Golpanian RS, Aickara D, et al. The effect of fatty acids, vitamins, and minerals on pediatric atopic dermatitis: A systematic review. Pediatr Dermatol 2023;40(1):44–9.

120. Senapati S, Banerjee S, Gangopadhyay DN. Evening primrose oil is effective in atopic dermatitis: a randomized placebo-controlled trial. Indian J Dermatol Venereol Leprol 2008;74(5):447–52.

121. KANEHARA S, OHTANI T, UEDE K, et al. Clinical effects of undershirts coated with borage oil on children with atopic dermatitis: A double-blind, placebo-controlled clinical trial. J Dermatol (Tokyo) 2007;34(12):811–5.

122. Zebda R, Paller AS. Phosphodiesterase 4 inhibitors. J Am Acad Dermatol 2018;78(3 Suppl 1): S43–52.

123. Yang H, Wang J, Zhang X, et al. Application of topical phosphodiesterase 4 inhibitors in mild to moderate atopic dermatitis: a systematic review and meta-analysis. JAMA Dermatol 2019;155(5):585–93.

124. Arcutis Announces positive results from INTEGUMENT-PED pivotal phase 3 trial of roflumilast cream 0.05% for the treatment of atopic dermatitis in children ages 2 to 5. News release. Arcutis; 2023. Available at: https://www.arcutis.com/arcutis-announces-positive-results-from-integument-ped-pivotal-phase-3-trial-of-roflumilast-cream-0-05-for-the-treatment-of-atopic-dermatitis-in-children-ages-2-to-5/. [Accessed 19 September 2023].

125. Eichenfield L. Efficacy and safety of roflumilast cream 0.15% in adults and children aged ≥6 with mild to moderate atopic dermatitis in two phase 3 trials (INTEGUMENT-1 and INTEGUMENT-2). S025. New Orleans, USA: AAD Annual Meeting; 2023.

126. Bissonnette R, Chen G, Bolduc C, et al. Efficacy and Safety of Topical WBI-1001 in the Treatment of Atopic Dermatitis: Results From a Phase 2A, Randomized, Placebo-Controlled Clinical Trial. Arch Dermatol 2010;146(4):446–9.

127. Peppers J, Paller AS, Maeda-Chubachi T, et al. A phase 2, randomized dose-finding study of tapinarof (GSK2894512 cream) for the treatment of atopic dermatitis. J Am Acad Dermatol 2019; 80(1):89–98.e83.

128. Dermavant reports positive topline results from ADORING 2 atopic dermatitis phase 3 trial of VTAMA® (tapinarof) cream, 1% once daily in adults and children as young as 2 Years old. News Release.

Dermavant; 2023. Available at: https://www.dermavant.com/dermavant-reports-positive-topline-results-from-adoring-2-atopic-dermatitis-phase-3-trial-of-vtama-tapinarof-cream-1-once-daily-in-adults-and-children-as-young-as-2-years-old. [Accessed 12 December 2023].

129. Dermavant reports positive topline results from adoring 1, the second atopic dermatitis phase 3 trial of VTAMA® (tapinarof) cream, 1% in adults and children as young as 2 years old. Business Wire. May 2023;16. Available at: https://www.businesswire.com/news/home/20230516005549/en/Dermavant-Reports-Positive-Topline-Results-from-ADORING-1-the-Second-Atopic-Dermatitis-Phase-3-Trial-of-VTAMA%C2%AE-tapinarof-Cream-1-in-Adults-and-Children-as-Young-as-2-Years-Old. [Accessed 16 May 2023].

Timing of Food Introduction and Allergy Prevention: An Update

Ami Shah, MD, Scott H. Sicherer, MD, Angela Tsuang, MD, MSc*

KEYWORDS

• Atopic dermatitis • Atopy • Diet diversity • Early introduction • Food allergy • Prevention

KEY POINTS

- Early introduction of peanut and egg, along with regular ingestion once introduced, should be encouraged for all infants starting around 6 months of age though not before 4 months to prevent the development of peanut and egg allergy, especially for those with severe atopic dermatitis because they are at highest risk for food allergy development.
- There is no evidence of harm with early introduction of other common food allergens within the first year of life, but more data are needed to determine if there is a specific benefit with early introduction of other foods.
- There is no evidence to support the use of hydrolyzed infant formulas to prevent the development of childhood atopy.
- Additional studies are needed to confirm potential protective benefit of infant diet diversity and maternal diet during pregnancy and lactation toward preventing food allergy or childhood atopy.
- Barriers exist with regards to practical implementation of guidelines of early allergen introduction for both physicians and patient's families.

INTRODUCTION

Food allergy prevalence has increased worldwide since the 1990s, with rates of peanut allergy having doubled to tripled in certain countries.[1] The development of food allergy is especially a concern for infants with moderate to severe atopic dermatitis.[2] Given the social, nutritional, and financial burden that accompanies a food allergy diagnosis, research efforts have focused on identifying practices that may prevent the development of food allergy. The Learning Early About Peanut (LEAP) trial was a landmark study that demonstrated that early and consistent ingestion of peanut in high-risk infants (defined as having severe atopic dermatitis, egg allergy, or both) aged 4 to 11 months could substantially reduce their risk of developing peanut allergy by 81% by 5 years of age, including in those infants who showed sensitization to peanut through skin prick testing.[3] These findings led to national and international professional organizations encouraging early introduction of peanut in high-risk infants. The National Institute of Allergy and Infectious Disease (NIAID) released addendum guidelines in 2017 to encourage early introduction of peanut in infants with mild to moderate atopic dermatitis around 6 months of age and to consider diagnostic evaluation before early introduction of peanut in infants with severe atopic dermatitis or an egg allergy by 4 to 6 months of age.[4] This was in stark contrast to guidelines published by the American Academy of Pediatrics (AAP) in 2000, which had recommended delaying introduction of common food allergens in high-risk infants until

Division of Allergy and Immunology, Icahn School of Medicine at Mount Sinai, One Gustave L Levy Place, New York, NY 10029, USA
* Corresponding author.
E-mail address: angela.tsuang@mountsinai.org

Dermatol Clin 42 (2024) 591–600
https://doi.org/10.1016/j.det.2024.04.003

toddlerhood.[5] The AAP recommendations had been rescinded in 2008 but did not espouse active early introduction of allergens, until an updated AAP report in 2019 incorporated early introduction of peanut.[6,7]

Since then, additional randomized clinical trials have investigated the role of early introduction of other allergenic foods to reduce the risk of food allergy. The Enquiring about Tolerance (EAT) study evaluated the effects of early introduction of 6 allergenic foods (cow's milk, peanut, cooked hen's egg, sesame, white fish, and wheat) between 3 and 6 months of age in breastfed infants from the general population compared with standard care (exclusively breastfed until 6 months of age followed by parental discretion of solid food introduction). Early introduction of allergenic foods led to a significant reduction of peanut (0% vs 2.5%, P=.003) and egg (1.4% vs 5.5%, P=.009) allergy in the per-protocol analysis compared with the introduction at 6 months of age.[8] There was no significant difference for cow's milk, sesame, white fish, and wheat.

In addition to the early introduction of allergenic foods into an infant's diet, other environmental and cultural factors may also play a protective role in food allergy prevention, which can be speculated based on the varying rates of food allergy found globally.[9] This article serves as an update to the article written by Gupta and Sicherer[10] and discusses data from prominent studies that have been published in the last 5 years regarding interventions to prevent food allergy development. Current guidelines on food allergy prevention and barriers to their implementation will also be reviewed. Of note, the relationship of food allergy as a trigger for atopic dermatitis is a separate topic and is discussed in a separate review.

SPECIFIC FOODS
Peanut

As mentioned earlier, the LEAP and EAT trials demonstrated strong evidence on the protective effect of early peanut introduction in high-risk infants and in infants from the general population.[3,8] After early introduction of peanut and regular ingestion for 5 years, this protective effect was maintained despite subsequently discontinuing peanut ingestion for 1 year.[11] However, when looking at the population level, an Australian study found no difference in the prevalence of peanut allergy after the successful implementation of the early introduction of peanut before 12 months of age.[12] In this study, 89% of infants were introduced to peanut by 1 year of age with a median age of introduction of 6 months.[12] Notably there were a higher number of infants of East Asian ancestry in the latter cohort. This could have impacted the overall result as these infants were found to have a higher likelihood of peanut allergy compared with Australian infants in a separate study.[13] When looking specifically at infants of Australian ancestry, early peanut introduction was associated with a lower risk of peanut allergy.[12]

Recent studies have focused on understanding the optimal timing and population for early peanut introduction. A team of international researchers developed predictive models using data from 4 different studies on early peanut introduction (LEAP screening and prevention, EAT, and Peanut Allergy Sensitization) and estimated that there would be a 77% reduction of peanut allergy at the population level when peanut was introduced to infants with atopic dermatitis at 4 months and infants without atopic dermatitis at 6 months.[14] This was much larger than the estimated reduction in peanut allergy when only infants with severe atopic dermatitis had early peanut introduction, which was thought to be less than 5%.[14] In addition, this group found that the estimated reduction of peanut allergy diminished with every month of delayed introduction, determining that if peanut introduction was delayed until 12 months for all infants, the prevalence of peanut allergy would decrease by only 33%.[14] Similarly, an observational study in the United States found that the odds of developing a peanut allergy increased for every month of delayed introduction and increasing severity of atopic dermatitis.[2] The findings from both studies suggest that the majority of children have developed peanut allergy by the first year of life, especially for infants with moderate to severe atopic dermatitis. Therefore, to effectively reduce the rate of peanut allergy at the population level, all infants need to be targeted at a younger age.[2,14,15]

Egg

There have been multiple randomized controlled trials on early egg introduction looking at different forms, frequencies, and amounts as previously summarized by Gupta and Sicherer.[10] A meta-analysis looking at data from 5 randomized clinical trials on early egg introduction found that introduction of egg between 4 and 6 months reduced the risk of egg allergy.[16]

Milk

In recent years, studies have been published looking at the effects of early cow's milk introduction. A randomized control trial conducted in Japan found through intention to treat analysis that infants from the general population who had frequent ingestion of cow's milk formula (at least 10 mL/day) between 1 and 2 months of age had decreased incidence of cow's milk allergy at 6 months of age (0.8%) compared with infants who strictly avoided cow's milk formula during that time frame (6.8%).[17] The median daily consumption of cow's milk in the ingestion group was 106 mL, which corresponds to approximately 1500 mg of cow's milk protein.[17] A subgroup analysis of these infants found that early discontinuation of cow's milk formula, especially before 1 month of age, was associated with a higher incidence of cow's milk allergy.[18] Similarly, a randomized control trial in Israel found that no infants who were fed at least 1 bottle of cow's milk daily for the first 2 months of life developed IgE-mediated cow's milk allergy while 0.85% of infants who were exclusively breastfed during that time frame did develop IgE-mediated cow's milk allergy.[19] Of note, infants who were assigned to the exclusively breastfeeding group were allowed supplementation with cow's milk formula, if needed. Post-hoc analysis found that the prevalence of IgE-mediated cow's milk allergy in this group was higher in those infants who were occasionally exposed to small amounts of cow's milk compared with those that had no exposure (3.27% vs 0.7%).[19] These results are supported by findings of observational studies that early (within the first 1–3 months) and ongoing ingestion of cow's milk can contribute to reduced risk of cow's milk allergy.[20–22]

However, other data suggest that introduction of cow's milk too early may not be beneficial. A different randomized clinical trial also conducted in Japan showed that infants who avoided cow's milk formula for at least the first 3 days of life and were instead supplemented with amino acid based elemental formula had decreased prevalence of cow's milk allergy at their second birthday compared with infants who were supplemented with at least 5 mL/day of cow's milk formula from birth to 5 months of age.[23]

While the data are somewhat conflicting, they suggest that if infants are supplemented with cow's milk formula early, these infants may benefit from having cow's milk exposure continue with some regularity and consistency. However, for breastfed infants who are not getting supplemental infant formula with cow's milk protein it may be beneficial to not consume this formula only occasionally but rather start products with cow's milk around 4 to 6 months as a regular part of the diet. Additional studies are needed to determine the exact timing and mechanism of cow's milk introduction to induce tolerance to cow's milk protein.[22]

Tree Nuts

There are a sparse number of published studies that have investigated early tree nut introduction. A longitudinal study in Australia (n = 2925) found that no child who had consumed cashew by their first birthday had a cashew allergy by 6 years of age, but 3.6% of children who had not eaten cashew by that time did develop a cashew allergy.[24] After adjusting for confounding variables, however, the finding was not determined to be statistically significant.[24] Randomized control trials are currently ongoing to determine the effects of specific and mixed tree nut introduction.[25,26]

Multi-food

The EAT study was the first randomized controlled trial to evaluate the impact of early introduction of multiple allergenic foods, including cow's milk, peanut, cooked hen's egg, sesame, white fish, and wheat.[2] As mentioned previously, a protective effect against development of only peanut and egg allergy was observed.[2] There was no difference noted in infant nutrition and breastfeeding rates compared with the rest of the population.[2] Since this study, the PreventADALL trial has looked at the effect of early introduction of multiple allergenic foods on food allergy development. The PreventADALL study was a multi-center randomized controlled trial that enrolled infants from the general population in Norway and Sweden and compared the development of atopic dermatitis and food allergy amongst 4 groups: (1) no intervention, (2) early complementary feeding of allergenic foods, (3) early skin emollient application, and (4) both food and skin interventions.[27,28] Early complementary feeding involved introducing peanut, cow's milk, wheat, and egg between 3 and 4 months of age and keeping the food in the diet at least 4 times a week until 6 months of age.[27] Participants in the trial developed peanut, egg, and cow's milk allergy, but not wheat allergy. Infants in the food intervention group had a decreased odds of food allergy development (odds ratio [OR] 0.4, 95% confidence interval (CI): 0.2–0.8) at 3 years of age.[27] When looking at individual foods, infants in the food intervention group had significantly decreased odds of developing peanut allergy (OR 0.4, 95% CI 0.2–0.8), but no significant difference was noted for egg or cow's milk allergy.[27]

DIET DIVERSITY

Diet diversity refers to the number of food or food groups consumed over a given reference period.[29] There has been a growing interest in understanding whether early infant diet diversity can be protective toward development of atopic disease, including food allergy. Analysis of a birth cohort study enrolling pregnant women from 5 European countries found that decreased diet diversity in the first year of life was associated with an increased risk of physician-diagnosed food allergy at up to 6 years of age.[30] However, this association lost statistical significance when taking reverse causality into account.[30] Data from a more recent birth cohort study looking at children born in the Isle of Wright found that increased diet diversity between 6 and 9 months significantly reduced the odds of food allergy diagnosis over the first decade of life.[28] More specifically, their analysis showed that for each additional food introduced by 6 months of age; the odds of developing food allergy in the first decade of life were reduced by 10.8% after adjusting for confounding factors.[31]

SKIN BARRIER

The dual allergen hypothesis suggests that infants with atopic dermatitis are at increased risk of food allergy because their impaired skin barrier allows for sensitization to food allergens through environmental exposure before these infants ingest these foods, thus bypassing the development of oral tolerance.[32] Recent studies have explored whether improving the skin barrier through early emollient application can reduce the risk of atopic dermatitis or food allergy. As mentioned earlier, the PreventADALL study compared the development of atopic dermatitis and food allergy in 4 groups: (1) no intervention, (2) early complementary feeding of allergenic foods, (3) early skin emollient application, and (4) both food and skin interventions.[27,28] The skin intervention consisted of petrolatum-based emollients applied to the body, ceramide-based cream applied to the entire face, and baths for 5 to 10 minutes with added emulsified oil at least 4 days per week from age 2 weeks to 8 months.[28] The skin intervention did not show any benefit toward reducing risk of atopic dermatitis by 1 year of age or food allergy by 3 years of age.[28]

A meta-analysis of 10 randomized control trials looking at prophylactic emollient application initiated within the first 6 weeks of life found no difference in the development of atopic dermatitis or food allergy sensitization.[33] Emollients used in the intervention arms ranged from creams, oils, gels, balms, and emulsions with varying regimens in terms of frequency and location of application.[33] Control arms were not prescribed any emollient regimen, but some studies did have skin care advice regarding bathing given to both

the intervention and control arms.[33] There was some protective benefit from atopic dermatitis development when emollients were used in high-risk infants (which were defined as having a strong family history of atopy) or were used continuously.[33] A Cochrane review analyzed data from 33 randomized controlled trials studying the effect of skin interventions in healthy infants less than 12 months of age without pre-existing food allergy, atopic dermatitis, or other skin condition. They found low to moderate certainty evidence that emollients are not effective in preventing atopic dermatitis and instead may increase the risk of food allergy and skin infection.[34]

MATERNAL DIET

There has been no benefit found from exclusion of allergenic foods from the maternal diet both during pregnancy and during lactation in the development of atopy. There has been interest in exploring whether the addition of allergenic foods or diverse food groups to the prenatal maternal diet can confer protection toward food allergy development in the child. Two systematic reviews and meta-analyses did not show any association between individual food or food groups in the maternal diet during pregnancy and subsequent childhood development of atopy.[35,36] Analysis of a birth cohort in Colorado found that maternal consumption of vegetables and yogurt during pregnancy were protective against development of allergic rhinitis, atopic dermatitis, and asthma up to age 4, while red meat, cold cereals, fried potatoes, rice or grains, and 100% fruit juice were associated with increased atopic disease.[37] However, these associations were not observed with the diagnosis of food allergy in this cohort.[37] For specific allergenic foods, there is an ongoing clinical trial in Australia looking to determine whether consumption of peanut and egg during pregnancy and while breastfeeding is associated with decreased diagnosis of peanut or egg allergy at 1 year of age.[38]

Similarly, there is little known about supplements in the maternal diet and the effect, if any, on child atopy. The meta-analysis performed by the European Academy of Allergy and Clinical Immunology (EAACI) found that regular supplementation with Vitamin D during pregnancy may reduce the risk of childhood diagnosis of asthma, but not atopic dermatitis or food allergy.[35] Another meta-analysis found that probiotic supplementation during late pregnancy may reduce the risk of atopic dermatitis in the infant, but not food allergy, based on data from 19 studies.[36] The investigators note, however, a positive association between probiotic supplementation and reduced cow's milk sensitization between ages 1 and 2 years.[36] In addition, this meta-analysis also found using data from 6 studies that fish oil supplementation may reduce the risk of egg sensitization (ie, positive tests for egg-specific IgE antibody), but not egg allergy or other food allergy or sensitization.[36]

BREASTFEEDING

While there are other health benefits of breastfeeding, there continues to remain no evidence of exclusive breastfeeding as a protective factor for development of food allergy. The meta-analysis looking at data from 260 published studies found no association between breastfeeding, exclusive breast-feeding, and the timing of solid food introduction during breast-feeding and food allergy diagnosis.[36] A few studies have explored the role of infant exposure to allergenic food protein through breast milk in preventing development of food allergy. Two studies found that the risk of sensitization to peanut was significantly reduced further when infants were not only introduced to peanut early, but their mothers also consumed peanut regularly while breastfeeding.[39,40] In both studies, a large percentage of mothers had a history of atopy. Further studies are warranted to determine if this protection can be seen in the general population and whether the reduced risk of sensitization correlates to reduced risk of development of food allergy.

HYDROLYZED FORMULA

Supplementation of hydrolyzed formula has not been shown to reduce the risk of atopy. A Cochrane systematic review and meta-analysis determined that short-term or prolonged supplementation with hydrolyzed formula does not confer any additional benefit toward prevention of allergic disease compared with supplementation with cow's milk formula.[41]

INFANT DIET SUPPLEMENTATION WITH VITAMIN D AND PROBIOTICS

It remains unclear whether infant diet supplementation with vitamin D and probiotics can play a role in atopy prevention. Clinical trials are currently ongoing regarding the effect of infant vitamin D supplementation on food allergy diagnosis.[42] No new data have been published regarding infant prebiotic or probiotic supplementation and its effect on development of food allergy, although clinical trials are underway.

CURRENT GUIDELINES

Since the LEAP trial, a burst of data from prominent studies informed national and international organizations to update recommendations on primary prevention of food allergy. The most recent update was a consensus document from the American Academy of Allergy, Asthma and Immunology, the American College of Allergy, Asthma, and Immunology, and the Canadian Society for Allergy and Clinical Immunology in 2020.[43] In terms of early introduction for specific foods, these guidelines recommend introducing peanut- and egg-containing foods to all infants starting around 6 months of age though not before 4 months. Once peanut or egg is introduced, it is advised that the food should be regularly maintained in the diet. High-risk infants are defined as those with severe atopic dermatitis while family history of atopy and the presence of a food allergy are stated to have "some increased risk". This distinction stems from publications that do not show a family history of food allergy as a risk factor to having clinically diagnosed food allergy.[2,44] In addition, no studies have demonstrated a pathophysiologic link between challenge-proven egg allergy and the development of other food allergy.[43] This is an important difference from previously published guidelines, which discuss using family history or presence of egg allergy to risk-stratify infants.[4] The consensus document guidelines also note that screening with skin prick testing or serum immunoglobulin (IgE) before home introduction is not required but can be considered based on shared decision-making with the patient and/or family. For the remaining allergenic foods, the workgroup advises not to delay introduction after an infant has started eating complementary foods at 6 months with similar recommendations regarding screening. **Table 1** provides the full list of recommendations from the workgroup. International guidelines provide similar guidance with slight variations. For example, the EAACI advises early introduction of peanut and egg in all infants between ages of 4 and 6 months, but does not provide guidance for early introduction of other allergenic foods.[45] In contrast, the Japanese Pediatric Guideline for Food Allergy does not recommend active introduction of any specific allergenic foods but advises against general delayed introduction.[46]

Barriers to successful implementation of early introduction of allergens have been recognized for both parents and physicians. In both the EAT and PreventADALL trials, adherence to feeding regimens as advised in the intervention arm was low, ranging from 24% to 44%.[8,27] The EAT study

Table 1
List of recommendations for primary prevention of food allergy through nutrition by the joint consensus of American Academy of Allergy, Asthma and Immunology, American College of Allergy, Asthma, and Immunology, and Canadian Society for Allergy and Clinical Immunology

Defining high risk	Consider infants with severe eczema at the highest risk of developing food allergy. Consider infants with mild to moderate eczema, a family history of atopy in either or both parents, or infants with one known food allergy potentially at some increased risk of developing food allergy (or an additional food allergy). Be aware that food allergy often develops in infants who have no identifiable risk factors. There is no evidence to clearly support the younger sibling of a peanut-allergic child is at increased risk of developing peanut allergy, though such infants may be at risk of developing peanut allergy secondary to delayed introduction of peanut.
Peanut	Introduce peanut-containing products to all infants, irrespective of their relative risk of developing peanut allergy, starting around 6 months of life, though not before 4 months of life. While screening peanut skin or sIgE testing and/or in-office introduction is not required for early introduction, this remains an option to consider for families that prefer to not introduce peanut at home; this decision is preference-sensitive and should be made taking into account current evidence and family preferences. Strongly consider encouraging either home introduction, or offering a supervised oral food challenge for any positive skin prick test (SPT) or sIgE result. Once peanut is introduced, regular ingestion should be maintained.
Egg	Introduce egg or egg-containing products to all infants, irrespective of their relative risk of developing allergy, around 6 months of life, though not before 4 months of life. Use only cooked forms of egg and avoid administering any raw, pasteurized egg-containing products. While screening egg skin or sIgE testing and/or in-office introduction is not required before early cooked egg introduction, this remains an option to consider for families that prefer to not introduce egg at home; this decision is preference-sensitive and should be made taking into account current evidence and family preferences. Strongly consider encouraging home introduction or offering a supervised oral food challenge for any positive SPT or sIgE result. Once egg is introduced, regular ingestion should be maintained.
Other allergenic foods	Do not deliberately delay the introduction of other potentially allergenic complementary foods (CM, soy, wheat, tree nuts, sesame, fish, shellfish), once introduction of complementary foods has commenced at around 6 months of life but not before 4 months. Before early introduction of these foods, screening skin or sIgE testing and/or in-office introduction is not required; however, the decision to screen or not is preference-sensitive and should be made by the clinician taking into account current evidence and family preferences. Strongly consider encouraging home introduction or offering a supervised oral food challenge for any positive SPT or sIgE result if screening is performed. Once introduced, regular ingestion should be maintained.
Diet diversity	Upon introducing complementary foods, infants should be fed a diverse diet, as this may help foster prevention of food allergy.
Hydrolyzed formula	Do not routinely prescribe or recommend the use of any HFs for the specific prevention of food allergy or development of food sensitization.

Maternal diet	We do not recommend maternal exclusion of common allergens during pregnancy and lactation as a means to prevent food allergy. We offer no recommendation to support any particular food or supplement in the maternal diet for the prevention of food allergy in the infant in either the prenatal period or while breastfeeding.
Breastfeeding	While exclusive breastfeeding is universally recommended for all mothers, there is no specific association between exclusive breastfeeding and the primary prevention of any specific food allergy.

Adapted from Azad MB, Dharma C, Simons E, Tran M, Reyna ME, Dai R, Becker AB, Marshall J, Mandhane PJ, Turvey SE, Moraes TJ. Reduced peanut sensitization with maternal peanut consumption and early peanut introduction while breastfeeding. Journal of Developmental Origins of Health and Disease. 2021 Oct;12(5):811-8.

team identified 3 main challenges that families faced with adherence, which were infant refusal of the food, concerns about reactions, and the practicality of incorporating this regimen into their daily lifestyle.[47] Other parental fears regarding early introduction, which were identified through survey studies, include concern for choking and lack of infant-safe forms.[48] Recent publications suggest that parental fears regarding safety may be warranted. An Australian study found that rates of food-induced anaphylaxis have increased in infants less than 1 year old since implementation of early introduction guidelines.[49] In addition, there has been an increase in non-IgE mediated food reactions such as food protein–induced enterocolitis syndrome, which is thought to be a consequence of early peanut introduction.[50] Finally, a retrospective chart review demonstrated an increase in peanut and tree nut aspirations since implementation of early peanut introduction guidelines in Australia.[51] In terms of concerns about practicality and availability of safe forms, commercial products in the form of powders, pouches, etc. containing either 1 or multiple allergenic foods have been developed to help make early introduction easier for families. These products, however, can be more expensive and may contain less food allergen compared with amounts used in research studies.[52,53] There

have also been reports of food reactions to the whole food (ie, peanut butter and scrambled egg) despite tolerating commercial products, which suggest that the amount of protein in some commercial products may not be enough to confer protection.[54]

Physician-identified barriers toward encouraging early introduction as noted through survey studies include perceived parental fear of reactions and parental lack of interest in early feeding along with lack of clinic time.[55] A survey conducted in New York suggested, however, that physicians may overestimate parental reluctance to introduce food allergens early.[48] Practical recommendations in terms of food preparation, dosing, and timing along with written materials to answer common parent questions have been developed to aid both physicians and patients' families with the adaption of early introduction guidelines.[43,53] In addition, a survey study found that the 2 most common reasons for deviations from guidelines by allergists were a family history of food allergy or positive skin prick testing.[55] The emphasis of the consensus document that family history is not considered a high-risk factor and that screening before introduction is not required (see **Table 1**) should hopefully assuage concerns previously held by physicians regarding for whom early introduction is appropriate.

Table 2
Environmental factors influencing in the development of food allergy

Risk Factors	Protective Factors	No Impact	Limited Literature
Severe atopic dermatitis	Early introduction of specific foods	Early skin emollient application	Infant vitamin D supplementation
Delayed introduction of peanut, egg	Infant diet diversity	Hydrolyzed formula	Prebiotics/Probiotics
	Maternal diet diversity	Breastfeeding	Maternal diet supplementation

SUMMARY

In the last 5 years, published studies continue to support the protective role of early allergen introduction in food allergy development. National guidelines now encourage early introduction of both peanut and egg for all infants starting around 6 months of age though not before 4 months and emphasize that screening with IgE testing is not required and may cause harm by unnecessarily delaying early introduction. Researchers have also identified other environmental interventions which may be beneficial in atopy prevention, including increasing infant and prenatal diet diversity. **Table 2** summarizes existing knowledge of the various environmental factors discussed in this article and their role in food allergy development. Randomized clinical trials are currently underway to better understand the impact that early introduction of other allergenic foods, maternal exposure to allergenic foods, infant vitamin D supplementation, and probiotic supplementation may have on food allergy and atopy development. In addition, research efforts should also be directed toward identifying mechanisms to address existing barriers that impede the practical implementation of early introduction of allergens in the United States.

CLINICS CARE POINTS

- Early introduction of peanut and egg, with regular ingestion once introduced, should be encouraged for all infants starting around 6 months of age though not before 4 months to prevent development of peanut and egg allergy, especially for those with severe atopic dermatitis as they are at highest risk for food allergy development. Pre-emptive allergy testing for those with severe atopic dermatitis or a known food allergy is optional but may be considered with shared decision-making.[43] Limited data exist regarding early introduction of other allergenic foods.

- Further studies are needed to demonstrate that infant and maternal diet diversity during pregnancy and lactation may be beneficial in prevention of childhood food allergy or atopy.

- Proactive emollient application within the first 6 weeks of life may not help prevent food allergy development.

- There is no evidence to demonstrate that use of hydrolyzed formulas helps to prevent development of atopy.

- Sparse data exist regarding the role of infant vitamin D supplementation, prebiotics or probiotics, and maternal diet supplementation on childhood atopy.

- Practical implementation of early allergen introduction has challenges identified by both patients' families and physicians.

DISCLOSURE

A. Shah has no financial conflict of interest to disclose. S.H. Sicherer reports royalty payments from UpToDate, Elsevier and from Johns Hopkins University Press; grants to his institution from the National Institute of Allergy and Infectious Diseases, United States, from Food Allergy Research and Education, United States, and from Pfizer, United States; and personal fees from the American Academy of Allergy, Asthma and Immunology as Deputy Editor of the Journal of Allergy and Clinical Immunology: In Practice, outside of the submitted work. A. Tsuang has no financial conflict of interest to disclose.

REFERENCES

1. Sicherer SH, Sampson HA. Food allergy: a review and update on epidemiology, pathogenesis, diagnosis, prevention, and management. J Allergy Clin Immunol 2018;141(1):41–58.
2. Keet C, Pistiner M, Plesa M, et al. Age and eczema severity, but not family history, are major risk factors for peanut allergy in infancy. J Allergy Clin Immunol 2021;147(3):984–91.
3. Du Toit G, Roberts G, Sayre PH, et al. Randomized trial of peanut consumption in infants at risk for peanut allergy. N Engl J Med 2015;372(9):803–13.
4. Togias A, Cooper SF, Acebal ML, et al. Addendum guidelines for the prevention of peanut allergy in the United States: report of the National Institute of Allergy and Infectious Diseases–sponsored expert panel. World Allergy Organization Journal 2017;10: 1–8.
5. American Academy of Pediatrics. Committee on nutrition. hypoallergenic infant formulas. Pediatrics 2000;106(2 Pt 1):346–9.
6. Greer FR, Sicherer SH, Burks AW. Committee on Nutrition and Section on Allergy and Immunology. Effects of early nutritional interventions on the development of atopic disease in infants and children: the role of maternal dietary restriction, breastfeeding, timing of introduction of complementary foods, and hydrolyzed formulas. Pediatrics 2008;121(1): 183–91.
7. Greer FR, Sicherer SH, Burks A, et al. The effects of early nutritional interventions on the development of atopic disease in infants and children: the role of maternal dietary restriction, breastfeeding, hydrolyzed

formulas, and timing of introduction of allergenic complementary foods. Pediatrics 2019;143(4):e20190281.

8. Perkin MR, Logan K, Tseng A, et al. Randomized trial of introduction of allergenic foods in breast-fed infants. N Engl J Med 2016;374(18):1733–43.

9. Warren CM, Turner PJ, Chinthrajah RS, et al. Advancing food allergy through epidemiology: understanding and addressing disparities in food allergy management and outcomes. J Allergy Clin Immunol Pract 2021;9(1):110–8.

10. Gupta M, Sicherer SH. Timing of food introduction and atopy prevention. Clin Dermatol 2017;35(4):398–405.

11. Du Toit G, Sayre PH, Roberts G, et al. Effect of avoidance on peanut allergy after early peanut consumption. N Engl J Med 2016;374(15):1435–43.

12. Soriano VX, Peters RL, Moreno-Betancur M, et al. Association between earlier introduction of peanut and prevalence of peanut allergy in infants in Australia. JAMA 2022;328(1):48–56.

13. Koplin JJ, Dharmage SC, Ponsonby AL, et al. Environmental and demographic risk factors for egg allergy in a population-based study of infants. Allergy 2012;67(11):1415–22.

14. Roberts G, Bahnson HT, Du Toit G, et al. Defining the window of opportunity and target populations to prevent peanut allergy. J Allergy Clin Immunol 2023;151(5):1329–36.

15. Bird JA. Please push the peanuts. J Allergy Clin Immunol 2023;151(5):1246–8.

16. Ierodiakonou D, Garcia-Larsen V, Logan A, et al. Timing of allergenic food introduction to the infant diet and risk of allergic or autoimmune disease: a systematic review and meta-analysis. JAMA 2016;316(11):1181–92.

17. Sakihara T, Otsuji K, Arakaki Y, et al. Randomized trial of early infant formula introduction to prevent cow's milk allergy. J Allergy Clin Immunol 2021;147(1):224–32.

18. Sakihara T, Otsuji K, Arakaki Y, et al. Early discontinuation of cow's milk protein ingestion is associated with the development of cow's milk allergy. J Allergy Clin Immunol Pract 2022;10(1):172–9.

19. Lachover-Roth I, Cohen-Engler A, Furman Y, et al. Early, continuing exposure to cow's milk formula and cow's milk allergy: The COMEET study, a single center, prospective interventional study. Ann Allergy Asthma Immunol 2023;130(2):233–9.

20. Peters RL, Koplin JJ, Dharmage SC, et al. Early exposure to cow's milk protein is associated with a reduced risk of cow's milk allergic outcomes. J Allergy Clin Immunol Pract 2019;7(2):462–70.

21. Natsume O, Yamamoto-Hanada K, Kabashima S, et al. Continuous cow's milk protein consumption from birth and a decrease in milk allergy: a prospective cohort study related to the PETIT study. J Allergy Clin Immunol 2018;141(2):AB85.

22. Abrams EM, Sicherer SH. Cow's milk allergy prevention. Ann Allergy Asthma Immunol 2021;127(1):36–41.

23. Urashima M, Mezawa H, Okuyama M, et al. Primary prevention of cow's milk sensitization and food allergy by avoiding supplementation with cow's milk formula at birth: a randomized clinical trial. JAMA Pediatr 2019;173(12):1137–45.

24. Peters RL, Barret DY, Soriano VX, et al. No cashew allergy in infants introduced to cashew by age 1 year. J Allergy Clin Immunol 2021;147(1):383–4.

25. McWilliam VL, Koplin JJ, Allen K, et al. TreEAT trial: Protocol for a randomized controlled trial investigating the efficacy and safety of early introduction of tree nuts for the prevention of tree nut allergy in infants with peanut allergy. Pediatr Allergy Immunol 2023;34(3):e13930.

26. Palmer DJ, Silva DT, Prescott SL. Feasibility and safety of introducing cashew nut spread in infant diets—A randomized trial. Pediatr Allergy Immunol 2023;34(6):e13969.

27. Skjerven HO, Lie A, Vettukattil R, et al. Early food intervention and skin emollients to prevent food allergy in young children (PreventADALL): a factorial, multicentre, cluster-randomised trial. Lancet 2022;399(10344):2398–411.

28. Skjerven HO, Rehbinder EM, Vettukattil R, et al. Skin emollient and early complementary feeding to prevent infant atopic dermatitis (PreventADALL): a factorial, multicentre, cluster-randomised trial. Lancet 2020;395(10228):951–61.

29. Ruel MT. Is dietary diversity an indicator of food security or dietary quality? A review of measurement issues and research needs. Food Nutr Bull 2003;24(2):231–2.

30. Roduit C, Frei R, Depner M, et al. Increased food diversity in the first year of life is inversely associated with allergic diseases. J Allergy Clin Immunol 2014;133(4):1056–64.

31. Venter C, Maslin K, Holloway JW, et al. Different measures of diet diversity during infancy and the association with childhood food allergy in a UK birth cohort study. J Allergy Clin Immunol Pract 2020;8(6):2017–26.

32. Lack G. Update on risk factors for food allergy. J Allergy Clin Immunol 2012;129(5):1187–97.

33. Zhong Y, Samuel M, van Bever H, et al. Emollients in infancy to prevent atopic dermatitis: a systematic review and meta-analysis. Allergy 2022;77(6):1685–99.

34. Kelleher MM, Phillips R, Brown SJ, et al. Skin care interventions in infants for preventing eczema and food allergy. Cochrane Database Syst Rev 2022;11(11):CD013534.

35. Venter C, Agostoni C, Arshad SH, et al. Dietary factors during pregnancy and atopic outcomes in childhood: A systematic review from the European

Academy of Allergy and Clinical Immunology. Pediatr Allergy Immunol 2020;31(8):889–912.

36. Garcia-Larsen V, Ierodiakonou D, Jarrold K, et al. Diet during pregnancy and infancy and risk of allergic or autoimmune disease: A systematic review and meta-analysis. PLoS Med 2018;15(2): e1002507.

37. Venter C, Palumbo MP, Glueck DH, et al. The maternal diet index in pregnancy is associated with offspring allergic diseases: the Healthy Start study. Allergy 2022;77(1):162–72.

38. Palmer DJ, Sullivan TR, Campbell DE, et al. PrEggNut Study: protocol for a randomised controlled trial investigating the effect of a maternal diet rich in eggs and peanuts from< 23 weeks' gestation during pregnancy to 4 months' lactation on infant IgE-mediated egg and peanut allergy outcomes. BMJ Open 2022;12(6):e056925.

39. Pitt TJ, Becker AB, Chan-Yeung M, et al. Reduced risk of peanut sensitization following exposure through breast-feeding and early peanut introduction. J Allergy Clin Immunol 2018;141(2):620–5.

40. Azad MB, Dharma C, Simons E, et al. Reduced peanut sensitization with maternal peanut consumption and early peanut introduction while breastfeeding. Journal of Developmental Origins of Health and Disease 2021;12(5):811–8.

41. Osborn DA, Sinn JK, Jones LJ. Infant formulas containing hydrolysed protein for prevention of allergic disease. Cochrane Database Syst Rev 2018; 10(10):CD003664.

42. Allen KJ, Panjari M, Koplin JJ, et al. VITALITY trial: protocol for a randomised controlled trial to establish the role of postnatal vitamin D supplementation in infant immune health. BMJ Open 2015;5(12):e009377.

43. Fleischer DM, Chan ES, Venter C, et al. A consensus approach to the primary prevention of food allergy through nutrition: guidance from the American Academy of Allergy, Asthma, and Immunology; American College of Allergy, Asthma, and Immunology; and the Canadian Society for Allergy and Clinical Immunology. J Allergy Clin Immunol Pract 2021;9(1):22–43.

44. Gupta RS, Walkner MM, Greenhawt M, et al. Food allergy sensitization and presentation in siblings of food allergic children. J Allergy Clin Immunol Pract 2016;4(5):956–62.

45. Halken S, Muraro A, de Silva D, et al. EAACI guideline: Preventing the development of food allergy in infants and young children (2020 update). Pediatr Allergy Immunol 2021;32(5):843–58.

46. Ebisawa M, Ito K, Fujisawa T. Japanese guidelines for food allergy 2020. Allergol Int 2020;69(3):370–86.

47. Voorheis P, Bell S, Cornelsen L, et al. Challenges experienced with early introduction and sustained consumption of allergenic foods in the Enquiring About Tolerance (EAT) study: A qualitative analysis. J Allergy Clin Immunol 2019;144(6):1615–23.

48. Lai M, Sicherer SH. Pediatricians underestimate parent receptiveness to early peanut introduction. Ann Allergy Asthma Immunol 2019;122(6):647–9.

49. Mullins RJ, Dear KB, Tang ML. Changes in Australian food anaphylaxis admission rates following introduction of updated allergy prevention guidelines. J Allergy Clin Immunol 2022;150(1):140–5.

50. Lopes JP, Cox AL, Baker MG, et al. Peanut-induced food protein–induced enterocolitis syndrome (FPIES) in infants with early peanut introduction. J Allergy Clin Immunol Pract 2021;9(5):2117–9.

51. Leung J, Ainsworth J, Peters R, et al. Increased rates of peanut and tree nut aspiration as a possible consequence of allergy prevention by early introduction. J Allergy Clin Immunol Pract 2021;9(8): 3140–6.

52. Filep S, Chapman MD. Doses of specific allergens in early introduction foods for prevention of food allergy. J Allergy Clin Immunol Pract 2022;10(1): 150–8.

53. Schroer B, Groetch M, Mack DP, et al. Practical challenges and considerations for early introduction of potential food allergens for prevention of food allergy. J Allergy Clin Immunol Pract 2021;9(1):44–56.

54. Cox AL, Shah A, Groetch M, et al. Allergic reactions in infants using commercial early allergen introduction products. J Allergy Clin Immunol Pract 2021; 9(9):3517–20.

55. Johnson JL, Gupta RS, Bilaver LA, et al. Implementation of the Addendum Guidelines for Peanut Allergy Prevention by US allergists, a survey conducted by the NIAID, in collaboration with the AAAAI. J Allergy Clin Immunol 2020;146(4):875–83.

Contact Allergy Screening for Atopic Dermatitis

Mykayla Sandler, BA[a], JiaDe Yu, MD, MS[a],*

KEYWORDS

- Atopic dermatitis • Contact allergy • Allergic contact dermatitis • Patch testing

KEY POINTS

- Atopic dermatitis (AD) and allergic contact dermatitis (ACD) involve separate immune pathways but often coexist.
- Patch testing (PT) is the gold standard in the diagnosis of ACD, and can be used to effectively identify ACD in patients with AD.
- Care must be taken when performing PT in patients with known or flaring AD to avoid eliciting an angry back reaction.

INTRODUCTION

Atopic dermatitis (AD) and allergic contact dermatitis (ACD) are common inflammatory skin diseases that present in both children and adults. Both involve separate immune pathways, and there is uncertainty in the literature regarding whether patients with AD have an increased or decreased risk of developing ACD. Nevertheless, recent studies demonstrate that AD and ACD can coexist and overlap clinically, posing a diagnostic challenge. In this review, we discuss the current evidence and guidelines regarding the screening for contact allergies in patients with AD.

BACKGROUND

Pathogenesis of Atopic Dermatitis

AD is a chronic inflammatory skin condition affecting 20% of children and 10% of adults.[1,2] AD is driven by a combination of skin barrier dysfunction, immune dysregulation, genetic predisposition, and environmental factors.[3–5] Mutations in the filaggrin gene are thought to be a key driver of disease in many patients, contributing to barrier disruption.[3,5,6] The inflammation in AD is predominantly driven by Th_2 dysregulation, along with Th_1, Th_{17}, and Th_{22} cells.[5] Involved inflammatory markers include IL-4, IL-5, and IL-13, among others.[4] Diagnosis of AD is generally clinical, with biopsy reserved for cases with an unclear diagnosis.[7] Treatment options include topical emollients, topical steroids, non-steroidal topicals (calcineurin inhibitors, PDE-4 inhibitors, and Janus kinase (JAK) inhibitors) and systemic immunomodulating therapies (dupilumab, JAK inhibitors, cyclosporine, and methotrexate).

Pathogenesis of Allergic Contact Dermatitis

ACD is a type IV delayed hypersensitivity reaction to an external antigen for example, furocoumarins in poison ivy. ACD presents as pruritic, erythematous patches, and plaques at the site of allergen contact.[8] It is estimated that at least 20% of the general population has a contact allergy.[9,10] While the pathogenesis is not yet fully understood, ACD reactions are composed of 2 phases: sensitization and elicitation.[5] In the sensitization phase during the first exposure to an allergen, antigen-presenting cells take up allergens in the skin and present them to regional lymph nodes, leading

[a] Department of Dermatology, Massachusetts General Hospital, Harvard Medical School, 50 Staniford Street, Suite 200, Boston, MA 02114, USA
* Corresponding author. Department of Dermatology, 50 Staniford Street, Suite 200, Boston, MA 02114.
E-mail address: jiade.yu@mgh.harvard.edu

Dermatol Clin 42 (2024) 601–609
https://doi.org/10.1016/j.det.2024.04.009
0733-8635/24/© 2024 Elsevier Inc. All rights reserved.

to the generation of antigen-specific T-cells. Then, in the elicitation phase, re-exposure to the allergen causes antigen-specific T-cells to be recruited to skin, causing inflammation.[5] ACD has traditionally been understood to be Th_1-driven, though the exact signaling pathway remains to be elucidated. A 2014 molecular profiling study demonstrated the immune polarization of contact allergens, showing that different allergens activate unique immunologic pathways, and suggesting that the pathophysiology of ACD is not homogenous.[11] Nickel was shown to primarily activate Th_1/Th_{17}, while fragrance was predominantly Th_2/Th_{22}.[11] ACD is diagnosed via patch testing (PT) and treatment involves allergen avoidance, along with topical and systemic immunomodulating treatments.[8]

Patch Testing

The gold standard of diagnosis for ACD is PT, which relies on the principle that an individual with a contact allergy will have a population of antigen-specific T-cells, derived during the sensitization phase of ACD.[12] Then, when the individual is re-exposed to the allergen, those T-cells will produce a clinically-evident local reaction at the direct site of exposure, corresponding with the elicitation phase.[12] During PT, panels containing sets of standardized or customized allergens are adhered onto the patient's skin (generally the back). The panels are removed after 48 hours, and the results are read 72 to 144 hours after application.[12] Exposure to the panels is intended to incite the elicitation phase for any existing contact allergens, thereby causing a local reaction at the site of the positive PT.[12] Positive contact allergens will appear as erythematous, edematous, vesicular, and/or eczematous plaques at the site of exposure.[12] This process is outlined by the International Contact Dermatitis Research Group (ICDRG).[13,14] PT can be customized with additional panels based on occupation and exposures, or with personal care products to increase the sensitivity of testing.

DISCUSSION
Relationship Between Atopic Dermatitis and Allergic Contact Dermatitis

While previously believed to be distinct entities given their unique pathophysiology, several studies have shown that the incidence of overlap of AD and ACD is quite high. A 2017 analysis of the Pediatric Contact Dermatitis Registry by Jacob and colleagues found that 30% of the 1142 included pediatric patients had concurrent diagnoses of both AD and ACD.[15] These children typically presented for PT at an earlier age and were more likely to have generalized dermatitis.[16] Additionally, a 2021 analysis of the North American Contact Dermatitis Group registry found that 20.7% of adults and 29.5% of children were diagnosed with both AD and ACD after PT.[17]

There is controversy in the literature regarding the pathophysiologic relationship between AD and ACD.[18] Early studies suggested that patients with AD had a higher elicitation threshold for positive contact allergens, and therefore a lower incidence of ACD, as compared to patients without AD.[18–21] However, the immune dysregulation, skin barrier dysfunction, and filaggrin mutations associated with AD are believed to be positively correlated with the development of ACD.[3,4] Additionally, the barrier disruption in AD has been shown to cause increased hypersensitivity to irritants and potentially allergenic chemicals.[3,6,22] Additionally, a 2016 study identified a link between Staphylococcus aureus infection and nickel allergy in patients with AD.[23]

A 2015 study used gene expression and immunohistochemistry to demonstrate that patients with AD had attenuated and differently polarized reactions to contact allergens, compared to those without AD, though the exact physiologic relationship is not yet fully understood.[24] Studies have shown that patients with AD may be less likely to react to strong allergens that initiate a Th1-driven response (such as neomycin and methylchloroisothiazolinone), but more likely to react to weak allergens that are predominately Th2-driven (such as propylene glycol or fragrances).[16,25] Finally, patients with AD are likely to use a variety of topical products, including moisturizers, calming soaps, antibiotics, and steroids, all of which may contain potential contact allergens, leading to sensitization and ultimately exacerbation of their dermatitis.[3,7,22,26]

The clinical data regarding the risk of ACD in patients with and without AD are also mixed. A 2017 meta-analysis investigating the risk for contact sensitization in patients with AD found no significant association between AD and contact sensitization, but noted that, in general population studies, ACD was more prevalent in patients with AD.[18] Additionally, a 2023 retrospective review of 912 children, 615 with AD and 297 without AD, found that children with AD were significantly more likely to have more than 1 positive PT result, compared to children without AD.[27] Some studies have also found higher rates of ACD in patients with nummular eczema.[3] It is therefore believed that the association between ACD and AD is complex, with many different relevant variables.[6]

Considerations in Diagnosis

While the exact pathophysiology connecting AD and ACD remains to be fully understood, it is known that the 2 conditions can coexist, and that they can be difficult to distinguish.[4,17] Both conditions can present with erythematous, pruritic patches, and plaques, and both may have an acute or chronic course.[27] In children and adults, the classic distribution of AD involves the antecubital and popliteal fossae, with hand and posterior neck involvement becoming more common in adulthood.[7] In infants, AD may present more on the face, trunk, and flexural surfaces.[7] ACD, on the other hand, presents at the site(s) of direct exposure to a contact allergen.[7] A high index suspicion for ACD much be maintained for children or adults with AD with unusual presentations and locations of involvement. The diagnosis of AD is generally clinical, while ACD is diagnosed via PT.[7,12] Histopathology often cannot distinguish between the 2, therefore biopsy is rarely indicated.[28]

Patch Testing in Patients with Atopic Dermatitis

The guidelines from a 2016 expert consensus opinion suggest the following indications for PT in patients with AD:[5]

- Dermatitis worsening or not improving with conventional AD therapy.
- Dermatitis that rebounds immediately after discontinuation of topical treatments.
- Distribution of dermatitis more consistent with ACD (head and neck, hands, feet, eyelids, perioral, etc).
- Therapy-resistant hand dermatitis in a working population.
- Adult-onset AD.
- Severe, widespread dermatitis before starting systemic immunosuppression.

PT is less likely to be useful in patients with classically distributed AD, long history of stable AD, or with well-controlled dermatitis with conventional AD therapies.[5]

PT is generally more difficult in patients with AD, especially in patients with active dermatitis.[29] Performing PT on already inflamed skin can lead to false positives and/or false negatives, and a concomitant ACD reaction can lead to flaring of underlying AD.[3] In patients with AD, PT is also complicated by an increased risk for irritant reactions that may be misinterpreted as positive allergic reactions.[5,6] Personal products used for AD may also cause PT irritant reactions, especially

if not diluted and applied properly.[5] On the other hand, patients who undergo PT during an AD flare may have a decreased contact sensitivity response, leading to false negatives.[6] Finally, patients with AD are more susceptible to climate-induced skin barrier changes, which can affect PT results.[5,30] For example, dry climates in the winter lead to increased transcutaneous water loss and xerosis, which are believed to have a greater effect on the rate of positive PT reactions in patients with AD compared to those without.[6,30] Both false positive and false negatives have the potential to interfere with a patient's treatment plan, treatment efficacy, and quality of life.

There are very few risks associated with PT, and reports of PT-associated severe allergic reactions including anaphylaxis are rare.[31] There is a theoretic risk that PT may sensitize patients to new allergens.[12] However, a 2006 review of 7619 patients with AD who underwent PT over a 14-year period found that less than 1% of patients were actively sensitized through PT.[32] Another potential risk in patients with AD is angry back syndrome, in which all of the PT sites become diffusely inflamed, making it difficult to discern true positive PT reactions (**Fig. 1**).[12] This is more common in patients with AD.

Contraindications to PT include severe dermatitis with no clear skin on which to test, or a history of severe allergic reaction to suspected allergens.[12] PT should not be performed over sites of

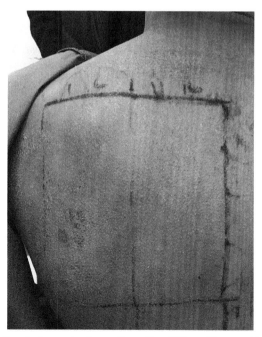

Fig. 1. Angry back reaction after PT in a 12-year-old child with severe AD.

recent or chronic topical steroid use, as this may lead to false negative results. Additionally, PT is typically performed in patients who are not using any systemic immunosuppressants.[33] However, more recent studies have shown that some systemic immunomodulators, especially when taken at low doses, do not significantly interfere with the results of PT.[5,34–36] It is therefore important to consider a patient's recent exposures and treatments when deciding whether to pursue PT.

Allergen Selection

During PT, patients are generally tested to a standardized allergen panel with or without additional, customized panels. There are currently over 30 available PT series, with some of the more common screening series being the American Contact Dermatitis Society (ACDS) Core Series (80 allergens) and the North American Contact Dermatitis Group Series (70 allergens).[12] Additional series are available based on relevant exposures, such as the cosmetic series, hairdressing series, and epoxy series, among others.[12] Allergen selection should consider a patient's occupation, hobbies, place of residence, and exposures based on the location of dermatitis.[3] Personal care products that come in contact with the location of dermatitis should also be included in testing.[3] In patients with AD, additional care should be taken to consider any topical treatments (prescriptions or over-the-counter emollients) that could serve as allergens.[5]

Allergen selection is particularly important when performing PT in very young children who have less surface area on which to apply patches.[37,38] Additionally, children and adults are known to have different contact allergen sensitization profiles, so it may not be appropriate or feasible to apply a 70 or 80-allergen panel onto a young child.[38–40] Children may not need to be tested to common occupational allergens, but rather testing should focus on allergens found in toys, play equipment, topicals, and antiseptics, among others.[37] In 2017, the Food and Drug Administration approved the Thin-Layer Rapid-Use Epicutaneous (TRUE) test to diagnose ACD in children above 6 years of age.[38,41,42] This test contains 35 allergens, and was meant to serve as a screening tool.[41,42] However, many relevant pediatric allergens were not included in this panel, and one study estimated that 39% of pediatric patients had a relevant positive PT reaction to an allergen not included in the TRUE test.[41,43] To address this discrepancy, members of the American Contact Dermatitis Society (ACDS) developed a standardized pediatric PT series by expert consensus in 2018.[38,44] This series contains 38 allergens and is intended to leave space for customization with additional patient-specific relevant allergens.[38]

Allergen selection for pediatric patients with AD becomes even more difficult when there is existing uncontrolled dermatitis on the back (**Fig. 2**), or when additional panels or personal care products must also be tested.[37] To address the issue of limited space for patches, providers may use the back, thighs, and abdomen, use smaller/limited pediatric series, or perform serial PT starting with the most high-yield allergens.[38]

Top Allergens in Patients with Atopic Dermatitis

Common allergens in patients with AD include fragrances, metals, surfactants, emollients, preservatives, plant-based mixes, and topical medications.[3,5,6,45,46] Several studies have investigated the top allergens in both children and adults with AD, with results summarized in **Table 1**.[15,17,27]

Fragrance

Fragrances are found in a vast array of products, including cosmetics, emollients, cleaning supplies, toys, and represent one of the most common allergens in patients with and without AD.[47,48] Common fragrance allergens to test to during PT include hydroperoxides of limonene and linalool, balsam of Peru, and fragrance mixes I and II.[3,48] Studies have shown an increased prevalence of contact allergy to fragrance in patients with AD.[47,49] If a patient tests positive to any fragrance, the recommended guidance is to avoid all fragrances as the current labeling standards in the United States do not require disclosure of specific fragrance allergens, making avoidance of specific fragrances impossible.

Metals

Metal allergy is common among patients with AD, particularly nickel and cobalt.[3] Nickel is a metal found in many different sources in today's environment, including jewelry, belt buckles, coins, toys, electronics, and razors.[16,50] Nickel can also be found in the water supply, as well as in certain foods. Nickel is currently one of the most common contact allergens in children and adults with and without AD, and guidelines have been published regarding the strict avoidance of skin contact with all nickel-containing objects.[16,43,51] Cobalt is also found in jewelry and belt buckles, as well as dental and orthopedic hardware.[16] It is also sometimes used as a color dye in porcelains, glass, paint, tattoos, leather goods, and hair dye.[16,52] Metal contact allergy may be particularly relevant to patients with hand dermatitis.[53]

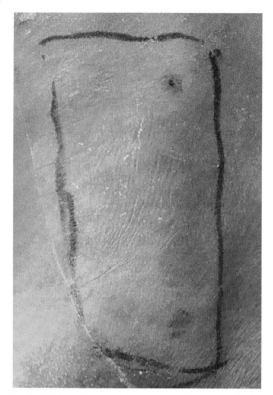

Fig. 2. PT in a 2-year-old patient with severe, flaring dermatitis on the back so that only 10 allergens could be applied.

Cocamidopropyl betaine

Cocamidopropyl betaine (CAPB) is a surfactant frequently found in shampoos and cleansers, particularly in products marketed for children.[16] CAPB was named the allergen of the year by the ACDS in 2004, due to its increasing prevalence in products.[54]

CAPB is one of the top contact allergens in children, and children with AD are estimated to have a significantly increased risk of developing a CAPB allergy, compared to those without AD.[15,16,55]

Lanolin

Lanolin is an oil-based wool extract found in many topical skin products and was given the dubious honor of the ACDS Contact Allergen of the Year in 2023.[16] Lanolin can be used as an emollient, moisturizer, emulsifier, adhesive, or plasticizer, making it a common ingredient in many products advertised toward patients with AD.[15,16] The exact composition of lanolin may differ based on source and processing, meaning that patients may react to some lanolin-containing products but not others.[15] Overall, the prevalence of lanolin allergy is believed to be increasing, and lanolin allergy has been shown to be significantly associated with a history of AD.[56,57]

Preservatives

Preservatives, including paraben mix, formaldehyde, quaternium-15, imidazolidinyl urea, diazolidinyl urea, DMDM hydantoin, and 2-bromo-2-nitropropane-1,3-diol (bronopol), among others, are commonly found in products such as emollients, topical steroids, and antibacterial creams.[58] Patients with AD may be exposed to these allergens in personal care products or topical treatments, and have been shown to be at increased risk of developing a contact allergy to formaldehyde releasers in particular, including quaternium-15, imidazolidinyl urea, DMDM hydantoin, and bronopol.[58] Overall, the rate of preservative contact hypersensitivity among adults with AD is estimated to be quite high; approximately 10% in 1 European study.[59]

Table 1
Top 10 allergens in children and adults with atopic dermatitis

| | Children | | Adults |
	Jacob et al,[15] 2017	Johnson,[27] 2023	Silverberg et al,[17] 2021
1	Nickel	Nickel	Nickel
2	Fragrance mix 1	MI	MI
3	Balsam of Peru	Fragrance mix 1	Formaldehyde
4	Bacitracin	CAPB	Fragrance mix I
5	Formaldehyde	Cobalt	Gold
6	CAPB	MCI/MI	Thimerosal
7	Propylene glycol	Hydroperoxides of linalool	Bacitracin
8	Wool alcohol	Formaldehyde	Cobalt
9	Lanolin	Balsam of Peru	Balsam of Peru
10	Bronopol	Amerchol L101 and Neomycin	Neomycin

Abbreviations: CAPB, cocamidopropyl betaine; MCI, methylchloroisothiazolinone; MI, methylisothiazolinone.

Compositae mix

Compositae are a family of plants, including ragweed, feverfew, dandelions, sunflowers, and daisies, which contain compounds called sesquiterpene lactones.[15] Exposure to compositae may occur from the environment or from skincare products.[16] Patients may react to one or all of sesquiterpene lactones, compositae mix, and dandelion extract.[16] In particular, children may be more likely to react to only dandelion extract, so this allergen should be tested specifically in children.[16,60]

Topical medications

Contact allergies to topical medications are quite prevalent and are estimated to affect 10% to 17% of those patients who undergo PT.[61] The most common medications causing ACD include topical steroids, topical antibiotics, local anesthetics, and nonsteroidal anti-inflammatory drugs.[61] These medications have also been found to be some of the top contact allergens in patients with AD.[3,15,16,62] While neomycin is one of the top allergens in both children and adults with and without AD, it remains unclear whether AD is a true risk factor for neomycin contact allergy.[63] Contact allergy to topical steroids is of particular concern in patients with AD, who may rely on these medications to control their disease.[62] Chronic inflammatory dermatosis and history of extended topical steroid use have been shown to be risk factors for developing contact allergy to topical steroids.[64,65]

Potassium dichromate

Potassium dichromate is a salt used in manufacturing, construction, leather processing, and pigments, among others.[15] Studies have shown that contact allergy to potassium dichromate is common among patients with AD.[3,15]

Propylene glycol

Propylene glycol is an emollient and emulsifier found in pharmaceuticals, topical therapies, cosmetics, fragrances and personal care products, among others.[3,66] Propylene glycol is a weak sensitizer, but acts as both an allergen and an irritant, confounding PT results.[66] Contact allergy to propylene glycol is common, but it remains unclear whether the risk of contact allergy is increased among patients with AD.[15,27]

SUMMARY

AD and ACD are common inflammatory skin diseases in both children and adults that present similarly and may coexist, posing a diagnostic and therapeutic dilemma. While the exact physiologic relationship between AD and ACD is poorly understood, the available evidence suggests that patients with AD have a unique inflammatory response to contact allergens and may react to different allergens than patients without AD. ACD is diagnosed via PT, and allergen avoidance is useful in the treatment of both AD and ACD. However, PT is more difficult in patients with underlying AD. Patients with AD may present with dermatitis on the back, decreasing the space on which to apply patches. This becomes more challenging in children, who have even less space on which to test. Additionally, patients with AD or severe ACD often require systemic immunosuppression, which may interfere with the mechanism of PT. Screening for contact allergens via PT is an important diagnostic and therapeutic tool for patients with recalcitrant AD, but must be done with caution, as testing may be complicated by the underlying disease pathophysiology.

CLINICS CARE POINTS

- AD and ACD are common inflammatory dermatologic conditions which may present similarly and may coexist, yet their treatments are distinct.
- PT is useful in the diagnosis of ACD and distinction from AD.
- Care must be taken when performing PT in patients with AD to avoid false positives or negatives.
- Identification of contact allergens via PT allows for allergen avoidance, which may be useful in the treatment of both AD and ACD.

DISCLOSURE

Dr J. Yu has served on the advisory boards for Arcutis, Sanofi, and Incyte; investigator for Abbvie, Sol-Gel, and Eli Lilly; consultant for National Eczema Association, O'Glacee, Edvyce; Board of Directors for American Contact Dermatitis Society and Pediatric Dermatology Research Alliance.

REFERENCES

1. Abuabara K, Ye M, Margolis DJ, et al. Patterns of atopic eczema disease activity from birth through midlife in 2 british birth cohorts. JAMA Dermatol 2021;157(10):1191–9.
2. Flohr C., Taieb A., French P.L., et al., Global Report on Atopic Dermatitis. 2022. Available at: https://www.eczemacouncil.org/global-atopic-dermatitis-atlas.

3. Owen JL, Vakharia PP, Silverberg JI. The role and diagnosis of allergic contact dermatitis in patients with atopic dermatitis. Am J Clin Dermatol 2018; 19(3):293–302.

4. Johnson H, Novack DE, Adler BL, et al. Can atopic dermatitis and allergic contact dermatitis coexist? Cutis 2022;110(3):139–42.

5. Chen JK, Jacob SE, Nedorost ST, et al. A pragmatic approach to patch testing atopic dermatitis patients: clinical recommendations based on expert consensus opinion. Dermat Contact Atopic Occup Drug 2016;27(4):186–92.

6. Thyssen JP, McFadden JP, Kimber I. The multiple factors affecting the association between atopic dermatitis and contact sensitization. Allergy 2014; 69(1):28–36.

7. Weidinger S, Novak N. Atopic dermatitis. Lancet 2016;387(10023):1109–22.

8. Brites GS, Ferreira I, Sebastião AI, et al. Allergic contact dermatitis: From pathophysiology to development of new preventive strategies. Pharmacol Res 2020;162:105282.

9. Alinaghi F, Bennike NH, Egeberg A, et al. Prevalence of contact allergy in the general population: A systematic review and meta-analysis. Contact Dermatitis 2019;80(2):77–85.

10. Adler BL, DeLeo VA. Allergic Contact Dermatitis. JAMA Dermatol 2021;157(3):364.

11. Dhingra N, Shemer A, Correa da Rosa J, et al. Molecular profiling of contact dermatitis skin identifies allergen-dependent differences in immune response. J Allergy Clin Immunol 2014;134(2):362–72.

12. Garg V, Brod B, Gaspari AA. Patch testing: Uses, systems, risks/benefits, and its role in managing the patient with contact dermatitis. Clin Dermatol 2021;39(4):580–90.

13. Lachapelle JM, Maibach HI. Patch testing and prick testing. Cham, Switzerland: Springer; 2012.

14. Fregert S. Manual of contact dermatitis: on behalf of the international contact dermatitis research group. Copenhagen: Munksgaard; 1974.

15. Jacob SE, McGowan M, Silverberg NB, et al. Pediatric contact dermatitis registry data on contact allergy in children with atopic dermatitis. JAMA Dermatol 2017;153(8):765–70.

16. Borok J, Matiz C, Goldenberg A, et al. Contact dermatitis in atopic dermatitis children—past, present, and future. Clin Rev Allergy Immunol 2019; 56(1):86–98.

17. Silverberg JI, Hou A, Warshaw EM, et al. Prevalence and trend of allergen sensitization in adults and children with atopic dermatitis referred for patch testing, north american contact dermatitis group data, 2001-2016. J Allergy Clin Immunol Pract 2021;9(7): 2853–66.e14.

18. Hamann CR, Hamann D, Egeberg A, et al. Association between atopic dermatitis and contact sensitization: a systematic review and meta-analysis. J Am Acad Dermatol 2017;77(1):70–8.

19. Uehara M, Sawai T. A longitudinal study of contact sensitivity in patients with atopic dermatitis. Arch Dermatol 1989;125(3):366–8.

20. Jones HE, Lewis CW, McMarlin SL. Allergic contact sensitivity in atopic dermatitis. Arch Dermatol 1973; 107(2):217–22.

21. Rystedt I. Atopic background in patients with occupational hand eczema. Contact Dermatitis 1985; 12(5):247–54.

22. Halling-Overgaard AS, Kezic S, Jakasa I, et al. Skin absorption through atopic dermatitis skin: a systematic review. Br J Dermatol 2017;177(1):84–106.

23. Bogdali AM, Grazyna A, Wojciech D, et al. Nickel allergy and relationship with Staphylococcus aureus in atopic dermatitis. J Trace Elem Med Biol Organ Soc Miner Trace Elem GMS 2016;33:1–7.

24. Correa da Rosa J, Malajian D, Shemer A, et al. Patients with atopic dermatitis have attenuated and distinct contact hypersensitivity responses to common allergens in skin. J Allergy Clin Immunol 2015; 135(3):712–20.

25. Kohli N, Nedorost S. Inflamed skin predisposes to sensitization to less potent allergens. J Am Acad Dermatol 2016;75(2):312–7.e1.

26. Rastogi S, Patel KR, Singam V, et al. Allergic contact dermatitis to personal care products and topical medications in adults with atopic dermatitis. J Am Acad Dermatol 2018;79(6):1028–33.e6.

27. Johnson H, Aquino MR, Snyder A, et al. Prevalence of allergic contact dermatitis in children with and without atopic dermatitis: A multicenter retrospective case-control study. J Am Acad Dermatol 2023. https://doi.org/10.1016/j.jaad.2023.06.048. S0190962223012707.

28. Frings VG, Böer-Auer A, Breuer K. Histomorphology and immunophenotype of eczematous skin lesions revisited-skin biopsies are not reliable in differentiating allergic contact dermatitis, irritant contact dermatitis, and atopic dermatitis. Am J Dermatopathol 2018;40(1):7–16.

29. Milam EC, Jacob SE, Cohen DE. Contact dermatitis in the patient with atopic dermatitis. J Allergy Clin Immunol Pract 2019;7(1):18–26.

30. Elias PM, Hatano Y, Williams ML. Basis for the barrier abnormality in atopic dermatitis: Outside-inside-outside pathogenic mechanisms. J Allergy Clin Immunol 2008;121(6):1337–43.

31. Daftary K, Scheman A, Bai H, et al. Rate of patch testing induced anaphylaxis. Dermat Contact Atopic Occup Drug 2023;34(1):33–5.

32. Jensen CD, Paulsen E, Andersen KE. Retrospective evaluation of the consequence of alleged patch test sensitization. Contact Dermatitis 2006;55(1):30–5.

33. Fowler JF, Maibach HI, Zirwas M, et al. Effects of immunomodulatory agents on patch testing: expert

opinion 2012. Dermat Contact Atopic Occup Drug 2012;23(6):301–3.

34. Rosmarin D, Gottlieb AB, Asarch A, et al. Patch-testing while on systemic immunosuppressants. Dermat Contact Atopic Occup Drug 2009;20(5): 265–70.

35. Mufti A, Lu JD, Sachdeva M, et al. Patch testing during immunosuppressive therapy: a systematic review. Dermat Contact Atopic Occup Drug 2021; 32(6):365–74.

36. Wentworth AB, Davis MDP. Patch testing with the standard series when receiving immunosuppressive medications. Dermat Contact Atopic Occup Drug 2014;25(4):195–200.

37. Johansen JD, Aalto-Korte K, Agner T, et al. European society of contact dermatitis guideline for diagnostic patch testing – recommendations on best practice. Contact Dermatitis 2015;73(4): 195–221.

38. Neale H, Garza-Mayers AC, Tam I, et al. Pediatric allergic contact dermatitis. Part 2: Patch testing series, procedure, and unique scenarios. J Am Acad Dermatol 2021;84(2):247–55.

39. Francuzik W, Geier J, Schubert S, et al. A case-control analysis of skin contact allergy in children and adolescents. Pediatr Allergy Immunol Off Publ Eur Soc Pediatr Allergy Immunol 2019;30(6): 632–7.

40. Brod BA, Treat JR, Rothe MJ, et al. Allergic contact dermatitis: Kids are not just little people. Clin Dermatol 2015;33(6):605–12.

41. Sindle A, Jacob S, Martin K. Common allergens and considerations when performing pediatric patch testing. Dermatol Clin 2020;38(3). https://doi.org/ 10.1016/j.det.2020.02.003.

42. U.S. Food and Drug Administration Center for Biologics Evaluation and Research. T.R.U.E. TEST Approval Letter. 2017. Available at: https://www.fda. gov/vaccines-blood-biologics/allergenics/true-test. [Accessed 14 November 2023].

43. Zug KA, McGinley-Smith D, Warshaw EM, et al. Contact allergy in children referred for patch testing: North American Contact Dermatitis Group data, 2001-2004. Arch Dermatol 2008;144(10): 1329–36.

44. Yu J, Atwater AR, Brod B, et al. Pediatric baseline patch test series: pediatric contact dermatitis workgroup. Dermat Contact Atopic Occup Drug 2018; 29(4):206–12.

45. Heine G, Schnuch A, Uter W, et al. Type-IV sensitization profile of individuals with atopic eczema: results from the Information network of departments of dermatology (IVDK) and the German contact dermatitis research group (DKG). Allergy 2006; 61(5):611–6.

46. Mailhol C, Lauwers-Cances V, Rancé F, et al. Prevalence and risk factors for allergic contact dermatitis to topical treatment in atopic dermatitis: a study in 641 children. Allergy 2009;64(5):801–6.

47. Thyssen JP, Linneberg A, Engkilde K, et al. Contact sensitization to common haptens is associated with atopic dermatitis: new insight. Br J Dermatol 2012; 166(6):1255–61.

48. De Groot AC. Fragrances: contact allergy and other adverse effects. Dermatitis 2020;31(1):13–35.

49. Thyssen JP, Johansen JD, Linneberg A, et al. The association between contact sensitization and atopic disease by linkage of a clinical database and a nationwide patient registry. Allergy 2012; 67(9):1157–64.

50. Fenner J, Hadi A, Yeh L, et al. Hidden risks in toys: A systematic review of pediatric toy contact dermatitis. Contact Dermatitis 2020;82(5):265–71.

51. Silverberg NB, Pelletier JL, Jacob SE, et al. Nickel allergic contact dermatitis: identification, treatment, and prevention. Pediatrics 2020;145(5):e20200628.

52. Fowler JF. Cobalt. Dermat Contact Atopic Occup Drug 2016;27(1):3–8.

53. Pootongkam S, Nedorost S. Allergic contact dermatitis in atopic dermatitis. Curr Treat Options Allergy 2014;1(4):329–36.

54. Jacob SE, Amini S. Cocamidopropyl betaine. Dermat Contact Atopic Occup Drug 2008;19(3):157–60.

55. Jacob SE, Yang A, Herro E, et al. Contact allergens in a pediatric population. J Clin Aesthetic Dermatol 2010;3(10):29–35.

56. Fransen M, Overgaard LEK, Johansen JD, et al. Contact allergy to lanolin: temporal changes in prevalence and association with atopic dermatitis. Contact Dermatitis 2018;78(1):70–5.

57. Warshaw EM, Nelsen DD, Maibach HI, et al. Positive patch test reactions to lanolin: cross-sectional data from the north american contact dermatitis group, 1994 to 2006. Dermat Contact Atopic Occup Drug 2009;20(2):79–88.

58. Shaughnessy CN, Malajian D, Belsito DV. Cutaneous delayed-type hypersensitivity in patients with atopic dermatitis: reactivity to topical preservatives. J Am Acad Dermatol 2014;70(1):102–7.

59. Németh D, Temesvári E, Holló P, et al. Preservative contact hypersensitivity among adult atopic dermatitis patients. Life 2022;12(5):715.

60. Paulsen E, Andersen KE. Sensitization patterns in Compositae-allergic patients with current or past atopic dermatitis. Contact Dermatitis 2013;68(5): 277–85.

61. de Groot A. Allergic contact dermatitis from topical drugs: an overview. Dermatitis 2021;32(4):197–213.

62. Kot M, Bogaczewicz J, Krecisz B, et al. Contact hypersensitivity to haptens of the European standard series and corticosteroid series in the population of adolescents and adults with atopic dermatitis. Dermat Contact Atopic Occup Drug 2014;25(2):72–6.

63. Gehrig KA, Warshaw EM. Allergic contact dermatitis to topical antibiotics: Epidemiology, responsible allergens, and management. J Am Acad Dermatol 2008;58(1):1–21.

64. Vind-Kezunovic D, Johansen JD, Carlsen BC. Prevalence of and factors influencing sensitization to corticosteroids in a Danish patch test population. Contact Dermatitis 2011;64(6):325–9.

65. Kot M, Bogaczewicz J, Kręcisz B, et al. Contact allergy in the population of patients with chronic inflammatory dermatoses and contact hypersensitivity to corticosteroids. Adv Dermatol Allergol Dermatol Alergol 2017;34(3):253–9.

66. Jacob SE, Scheman A, McGowan MA. Propylene glycol. Dermat Contact Atopic Occup Drug 2018; 29(1):3–5.

Special Considerations in Atopic Dermatitis in Young Children

Mudra Bhatt, MBBS[a], Karan Lal, DO MS[b,c], Nanette B. Silverberg, MD[d,*]

KEYWORDS

- Atopic dermatitis • Vaccination • Teething • Dupilumab • Comorbidities

KEY POINTS

- The comorbidities of atopic dermatitis in early childhood include allergic phenotypes as seen in the atopic march, dry skin, ophthalmologic findings, infectious, psychiatric, and comorbid skin diseases.
- Although it is not completely proven, the availability of more options and earlier disease control are expected to result in less severe disease overtime.
- Vaccination, growth and development, tactile sensation development, and facial skin care during teething represent specific age-based challenges in children under the age of 2 years.

INTRODUCTION

Atopic dermatitis (AD) is a common inflammatory skin condition associated with genetic and environmental factors that trigger onset. Eighty percent of cases occur before the age of 6 years, 60% in the first 12 months of life,[1] and the lifetime prevalence of AD in children ages 3 to 11 years is 20%.[1] Consequently, early childhood disease, that is, AD before the age of 6 years, is important, not only due to incidence, but also due to the early interventions that could modify lifetime risk of comorbidities and AD disease severity.

TRIGGERS

A recent hospital-based study addressed triggers for AD in young children. These included neonatal hyperbilirubinemia, neonatal respiratory distress syndrome, neonatal infection, and infection during childhood, all of which had effect on onset of symptoms and persistence in early childhood (until age 5 years).[2] Immunoglobulin E (IgE) levels were also raised by neonatal respiratory distress syndrome (NRDS) and neonatal hyperbilirubinemia, with contribution to disease activity in that population.[2] *Malassezia* overgrowth (ie, seborrheic dermatitis), although the mechanism for this is not fully elucidated, has been linked to onset and aggravation of AD.[3] Seborrheic dermatitis (cradle cap) is very common in young children, and this may be considered the herald of new-onset AD for many young kids. Molluscum contagiosum infections have been associated with new-onset AD, particularly in the popliteal area, for children aged under 5 years, and flaring of existent AD.[4]

PRESENTATION

The cardinal features of AD are itching that is often referred to as "itch that rashes" and dryness of the skin.[5,6] Atopic stigmata are typical skin signs, not pathologic themselves, that indicate an atopic diathesis. These include dry skin, hyperlinearity of the palms and soles, infraorbital double eyelid crease, periorbital halo formation, facial pallor,

[a] Government Medical College, Bhavnagar, India; [b] Affiliated Dermatology, Scottsdale, AZ, USA; [c] Department of Dermatology, Northwell Health, 101 Saint Andrews Lane Floor 1, Glen Cove, NY 11542, USA; [d] Department of Dermatology, Icahn School of Medicine at Mount Sinai, 5 East 98th Street, New York, NY 10028, USA
* Corresponding author.
E-mail address: drsilverberg@yahoo.com

Dermatol Clin 42 (2024) 611–617
https://doi.org/10.1016/j.det.2024.05.003
0733-8635/24/© 2024 Elsevier Inc. All rights reserved, including those for text and data mining, AI training, and similar technologies.

rarefaction of the lateral portion of the eyebrow, and white dermographism.[7]

The first consensus-based definition of AD was collated by Hanifin and Rajka in their seminal work.[8] The clinical features included 4 major criteria: pruritus, which remains a universal feature, typical morphology and distribution which we will review later as it pertains to different racial/ethnic differences in early childhood, chronic relapsing course, and personal/family history of atopy. The minor features included a list of 16 clinical parameters, many of which addressed life-course and co-morbid disease in children with early-onset AD. Therefore, we do not see many of these criteria in early childhood. The presentation and specific criteria noted in early childhood have been addressed in multiple studies worldwide. In addition to pruritic dermatitis, features of xerosis (xerosis, Dennie–Morgan folds, hyperlinearity, ichthyosis vulgaris, keratosis pilaris, white dermographism), and sensitivity (environmental aggravation, wool intolerance) lead to symptoms early on, but tendency to infections becomes prevalent in early childhood. Association of AD with upper respiratory infections, warts, molluscum, and *Strep* pharyngitis has been reported. Some atopic locations are notably more common for younger children. In China, eyelid dermatitis (49.8%), retroauricular/infra-auricular fissures (44.8%), and scalp dermatitis (49.7%) were more common in infantile patients with AD. Asthma became increasingly more common with age, while food allergies had the greatest prevalence in younger children and reduced with time.[9] While not as frequent, scalp dermatitis and ear fissuring were also recorded by Wahab and colleagues highlighting these features in Asian children worldwide.[10] Persistent disease has been noted to have a negative effect on early-childhood height and weight.[2] In India, 95% of children with AD present with xerosis and 55% with pityriasis alba, highlighting pigmentation as an important form of AD in children.[11] Xerosis is noted in 100% of children from Sweden.[12] Dennie–Morgan folds affected 80% of children in that study. In Bangladesh, studies of childhood AD highlighted xerotic features including hyperlinearity, ichthyosis vulgaris, and keratosis pilaris and a tendency toward cutaneous infections in 80%.[10] Hyperlinearity was seen in almost half of children from Thailand supporting this as a frequent feature in Asian children.[13]

In the Copenhagen Prospective Study on Asthma in Childhood, involving pregnant women with a history of asthma and infants during the first month of age, it was found that the progression of skin region involvement in infants who develop AD begins on the scalp, forehead, ear, and neck in a Balaclava-like pattern, continuing to the extensor sides and trunk, finally affecting the flexor sides of the extremities.[14]

In fair-skinned children, variants of dermatitis favor erythematous, oozing plaques, which may become lichenified with time and feature excoriations. In darker skinned children, erythema is often obscured by baseline pigmentation. This results in violaceous lesions, prominence of hyperpigmentation, and follicular variants of AD wherein the hair follicles become prominent with overlying extremely pruritic papules. A recent study from Genoa focusing on AD in children of color noted intense xerosis, xerosis-related features such as nummular eczema, prurigo nodularis-type lesions, and extensor site eczema as specific to kids of color.[15] Other variants that vary in darker skinned children include more frequent presence of nummular variants, lower rates of patch testing referral, and delays in therapy with lower access to care that is associated with greater usage of emergency room visits, and greater disease severity in black and Hispanic children in the United States.[16–19] In fact, on highly pigmented skin, the characteristic erythema appears gray ("ashy") or dark brown rather than red as in Caucasians.[7,20,21]

One difficult-to-treat situation of AD is the combination with irritant contact dermatitis of the face. This type is associated with extensive open, weeping lesions of the skin of the cheeks, chin, and upper chest where copious saliva produced in response to teething will land. Additionally, messy eating contributes to ongoing irritation. Management often includes frequent barrier-emollient application, reduced harsh cleansing, and sometimes preventive dosing of nonsteroidal or steroidal agents.[22] Once teething completes, the facial irritation abates.

MEDICATIONS FOR CHILDREN UNDER THE AGE OF 5 YEARS INCLUDING DIFFERENCES IN ABSORPTION BASED ON BODY SURFACE AREA

Specific considerations affect our choice of medications in early childhood. Specifically, there is a higher body surface area (BSA)-to-weight ratio that results in concern for greater absorption and risk of adverse events.[23] While most children have reduced absorption of drugs through the skin as their skin disease and barrier improve in tandem with AD therapy, some children have intrinsic barrier defects and continue to absorb drug. This is particularly true for children with Netherton syndrome and lamellar ichthyosis, whose skin barrier results in continuous absorption of drug. For these children, care and caution in usage of medications are needed particularly with the usage of topical tacrolimus that can have increased detectable blood levels when used in these conditions.[24]

Growth and development are important and rapid in early childhood. There are multiple concerns about AD with respect to growth and development. Topical corticosteroids applied in a sustained manner over a large surface area and oral steroid pulses could interfere with growth.[25] Sleep disturbance could interfere with vertical growth and psychosocial development.[26,27] Having extensive skin lesions of AD may interfere with sensory development.[28] This latter issue can benefit from more aggressive therapies, referral for early intervention evaluations, and massage therapy.[29–31]

Many topical corticosteroids have US Food and Drug Administration (FDA) approval. Ultimately, topical corticosteroid safety and efficacy is often paradoxic. While we presume conceptually that weaker topical corticosteroid classes are safer, in fact, lesions often clear more efficiently with a stronger agent, resulting in less burden and less length of corticosteroid exposure. The first such study that looked at hydrocortisone 1% cream versus mometasone 0.1% cream in 48 children with AD noted that one child had hypothalamic–pituitary–adrenal (HPA) axis suppression in the hydrocortisone arm, and none in the mometasone arm.[32] In general in systematic review, higher potency topical corticosteroids (TCS) are more effective.[33] Usage of Class II–III TCS can be considered in younger children as a rescue medication for severe flares. However, severe AD and higher total BSA are associated with greater TCS side effects; therefore, we must be mindful of careful observation and the need for nonsteroidal holidays for individuals with large BSA.[34] Higher BSA and higher baseline severity are also associated with greater resistance to lower potency agents.[35] HPA axis suppression can occur in children up until 18 months of age with topical steroid use; thus, counseling about appropriate tapering is essential to prevent topical steroid withdrawal and unrealistic expectations about AD which is a chronic disease with an unknown prognosis in most children.

Crisaborole 2% ointment is FDA approved for AD in children aged 3 months and older twice daily for active disease and once daily for maintenance. In Canada, pimecrolimus 1% cream is approved for AD in the age of 3 months and older, while children under the age of 2 years receiving topical calcineurin inhibitors are off-label in the United States. Usage for sensitive skin regions is helpful to avoid skin thinning and ocular changes associated with TCS.[36] Both crisaborole and tacrolimus are well known for their stinging sensation upon application, but this does improve usually after 2 weeks of use. Preemptive counseling can avoid noncompliance.

Dupilumab

Dupilumab is FDA approved for children with moderate-to-severe AD who have failed standard therapy for ages 6 months and over with a sliding scale dose based on weight and age. In recent studies discussing attenuation of atopic march, in a population with inadequately controlled AD, dupilumab significantly reduced new/worsened allergic events versus placebo. Persistent, attenuated effects, with remarkable reduction in serum total IgE levels, were observed even after discontinuing dupilumab therapy in off-treatment periods, with no rebound in allergic events, as evidenced by continued treatment benefits in follow-up periods after discontinuation of therapy. Greater impact was observed in the white population when compared to Asian population, likely due to larger number of baseline allergies in Caucasians.[37] Dupilumab is meant to be a chronic treatment which in itself requires a thorough discussion to reduce the risk of interruption and therapy and risk of inefficacy upon drug retrial. As such a vaccination plan has to be made in many children, given that the drug was not tested concurrent with live vaccines.

Vaccination Efficacy and Safety During Therapeutic Care of Children with Atopic Dermatitis

Vaccinations stimulate adequate immune response in children receiving topical calcineurin inhibitors[38] and adults treated with dupilumab.[39] A panel of 5 experts published a consensus on usage of dupilumab with vaccination. They indicated that live vaccinations should be given, where possible, at least 4 weeks before dupilumab initiation. Inactivated vaccines did not require discontinuation of drug, and the panel suggested there was no AD-exacerbation risk with vaccination.[40] When patients have been on dupilumab, there are no data on live vaccine usage, and according to the expert-panel, avoidance of live vaccination is preferred.[40] Ultimately, if we are to believe that live vaccines are unsafe on dupilumab, a 12 week holiday may be needed as a washout period before live vaccination. However, data are emerging from children who do not heed advice and had measles, mumps, rubella vaccine (MMR) vaccine with or without varicella vaccine, some within the 12 weeks that should be waited.[41] The 9 children recently described in case series will need to be corroborated but support the possibility of trial of vaccination on dupilumab.

THE MEDICAL HOME FOR SMALL CHILDREN WITH ATOPIC DERMATITIS

The concept of the medical home is highly applicable to AD. Parents care for a child with chronic illness in their households. As a result, we have to provide parents with the prescriptions, over-the-counter (eg, emollients), and educational support they need to be able to fight the good fight on a daily basis.

Considerations for enhancing the efficacy of the medical home include

1. Having household contacts contributes to the child's health. All members of the household should avoid smoking and kissing the child with open cold sores. Additionally, household members should avoid the usage of agents that promote irritation, like wool and fragrance, which can worsen AD when worn by a caregiver carrying an infant
2. Provision of an eczema action plan[42,43]
3. Enrollment of parents in eczema schools, where applicable[44]
4. Provision of rescue medications for step-up therapy
5. Counseling on when to be concerned with skin symptoms, for example, fever and spreading blisters

INFECTIONS IN CHILDREN WITH ATOPIC DERMATITIS

As young children with AD are more prone to catch or have severe flares of infections overlapping their AD, it merits mention of recognition of infection-associated flares and management considerations. A child with active AD will often appear in a medical office with relation to infections every 2 to 4 years. Infections associated with AD start from early childhood with a particular propensity for *Staphylococcus aureus* overgrowth on untreated lesions, spanning to more extensive molluscum contagiosum virus (MCV) lesions in toddler to school-aged children, extensive viral exanthems with co-localization to areas of AD, folliculitis, and impetigo in school-aged children, and extensive warts in pre-teens and teens. Infections with co-localization include eczema coxsackium associated with Coxsackie infections, eczema herpeticum associated with cutaneous herpes simlex virus (HSV) infection, and Kaposi's varicelliform eruption. It is important to recognize eczema herpeticum and Kaposi's varicelliform eruption as they merit antiviral medications, and in some cases hospitalization. Because *S aureus* is so often sitting on the areas of AD, progression to bacterial infection often overlaps cutaneous viral exanthems that involve open ulcerations. Good clinical care reduces infectious spread, and in particular, immunomodulation with dupilumab may reduce number and severity of infections. We have had the clinical experience that AD children with frequent infectious admissions can stay out of the hospital if treated with dupilumab. A post hoc analysis of the LIBERTY AD PRESCHOOL trial demonstrated reduced bacterial infections for patients treated with dupilumab, with data being equivocal for herpes infections.[45] Good skin care including bleach bathes and topical corticosteroids have also been shown to reduce infections in young children with AD.[46,47] Newer therapies such as endolysins are being employed in the management of AD to downregulate *S aureus* growth with no concern for resistance.[48]

PREVENTION OF LONG-TERM COMORBIDITIES

Food allergy prevention is well addressed in 2 other articles in this issue, therefore, we will limit our comments to some data on the prevention of asthma and allergic rhinitis in small children. The Protection Against Allergy Study in Rural Environments is a European birth cohort study that reported 4 phenotypes of AD in childhood: 2 early phenotypes with onset before the age of 2 years, that is, early transient and early persistent, the late phenotype with onset at age 2 years or older, and the never/infrequent phenotype, defined as children with no AD. Both early phenotypes of AD showed a tendency of an increased risk of developing asthma or food allergy, although the association was stronger with the early-persistent phenotype. The proportion of children having asthma was 17.5% among children with early-persistent phenotype (n = 10) compared with 7.5% among those with never/infrequent AD (n = 55). Meanwhile, the late phenotype seems to be different, being only associated with allergic rhinitis and not with asthma or food allergy.[49] Certain studies have shown the potential protective effect of yogurt's consumption in the first year of life on physician diagnosis of AD and other allergic diseases,[50,51] with the current results showing that this protective effect of yogurt in the first year of life was only on the early-persistent phenotype of AD.[49]

One older study, the early treatment of the atopic child trial found associations of asthma with filaggrin loss of function mutations.[52,53] The treatment of toddlers with daily cetirizine halved the risk of asthma in children allergic to house dust mite or pollen.[53,54]

SUMMARY

Younger children are most likely to develop and live with AD. Their concerns in relationship to the diagnosis of AD should be harmonized with their growth, development, sleep hygiene, and general well-being. Considerations for optimizing skin care in children with AD include being mindful in differences based on race and ethnicity, good skin care habits including infection prevention, promotion of sleep, and prevention of comorbidities. Enhancing understanding of skin care and general health in younger children with AD requires a holistic approach to address the many facets of this multisystem inflammatory disorder.

CLINICS CARE POINTS

- Provision of care in young children with AD first requires careful recognition of all subtypes of AD and nuanced care to address skin morphologic changes.

- Education and support of the medical home in children with AD include a variety of educational tools including eczema school and eczema action plans.

- The opportunity may exist to intervene effectively with the younger child with AD immune system to positively prevent comorbidities, which may be conducted in collaboration with allergists.

DISCLOSURE

Dr Mudra Chatt has no conflicts to declare. Dr Karan Lal has the following conflicts; Incyte (speaker), Abbvie (speaker), Pfizer (speaker), Boehringer Ingelheim (speaker), Galderma (speaker), Aerolase (speaker), Sanofi (speaker). Dr Nanette Silverberg is an investigator of Avita, and advisor/consultant/ speaker for Avita, Incyte, Novan, Pfizer, Regeneron, Sanofi, and Verrica.

REFERENCES

1. Kay J, Gawkrodger DJ, Mortimer MJ, et al. The prevalence of childhood atopic eczema in a general population. J Am Acad Dermatol 1994;30(1):35–9. PMID: 8277028.
2. Song K, Zhang Y, Wang L, et al. Risk Factors of Onset Time and Persistence of Atopic Dermatitis in Children Under Age 5 Years: A Cross-Sectional Study. Dermatitis 2024;35(S1):S47–54. Epub 2023 Dec 22. PMID: 38133542.
3. Glatz M, Bosshard PP, Hoetzenecker W, et al. The role of malassezia spp. in atopic dermatitis. J Clin Med 2015;4(6):1217–28. PMID: 26239555; PMCID: PMC4484996.
4. Silverberg NB. Molluscum contagiosum virus infection can trigger atopic dermatitis disease onset or flare. Cutis 2018;102(3):191–4. PMID: 30372710.
5. Sathishkumar D, Moss C. Topical therapy in atopic dermatitis in children. Indian J Dermatol 2016;61(6): 656–61. PMID: 27904185; PMCID: PMC5122282.
6. Tollefson MM, Bruckner AL. Section on dermatology. atopic dermatitis: skin-directed management. Pediatrics 2014;134(6):e1735–44. PMID: 25422009.
7. Wollenberg A, Werfel T, Ring J, et al. Atopic dermatitis in children and adults—diagnosis and treatment. Dtsch Arztebl Int 2023;120(13):224–34. PMID: 36747484; PMCID: PMC10277810.
8. Hanifin JMRG. Diagnostic features of atopic dermatitis. Acta Derm Venereol (Stockh) 1980;92(suppl):44–7.
9. Shi M, Zhang H, Chen X, et al. Clinical features of atopic dermatitis in a hospital-based setting in China. J Eur Acad Dermatol Venereol 2011;25(10): 1206–12. Epub 2011 Jan 9. PMID: 21214635.
10. Wahab MA, Rahman MH, Khondker L, et al. Minor criteria for atopic dermatitis in children. Mymensingh Med J 2011;20(3):419–24. PMID: 21804505.
11. Shetty NS, Lunge S, Sardesai VR, et al. a cross-sectional study comparing application of Hanifin and Rajka Criteria in Indian Pediatric Atopic Dermatitis Patients to that of Other Countries. Indian Dermatol Online J 2022;14(1):32–7. PMID: 36776180; PMCID: PMC9910542.
12. Böhme M, Svensson A, Kull I, et al. Hanifin's and Rajka's minor criteria for atopic dermatitis: which do 2-year-olds exhibit? J Am Acad Dermatol 2000; 43(5 Pt 1):785–92. PMID: 11050581.
13. Wisuthsarewong W, Viravan S. Diagnostic criteria for atopic dermatitis in Thai children. J Med Assoc Thai 2004;87(12):1496–500. PMID: 15822547.
14. Halkjaer LB, Loland L, Buchvald FF, et al. Development of atopic dermatitis during the first 3 years of life: the Copenhagen prospective study on asthma in childhood cohort study in high-risk children. Arch Dermatol 2006;142(5):561–6. PMID: 16702493.
15. Herzum A, Occella C, Gariazzo L, et al. Clinical features of atopic dermatitis in pediatric patients with skin of color and comparison with different phototypes. Skin Res Technol 2024;30(2):e13614.
16. Luu M, Diaz LZ, Chiu YE, et al. Pediatric atopic dermatitis: assessment of burden based on lesional morphology. PeDRA 2022.
17. Mitchell KN, Tay YK, Heath CR, et al. Review article: Emerging issues in pediatric skin of color, Part 2. Pediatr Dermatol 2021;38(Suppl 2):30–6. Epub 2021 Oct 27. PMID: 34708446.
18. Silverberg JI, Vakharia PP, Chopra R, et al. Phenotypical differences of childhood- and adult-onset

atopic dermatitis. J Allergy Clin Immunol Pract 2018; 6(4):1306–12. Epub 2017 Nov 10. PMID: 29133223; PMCID: PMC5945342.

19. Kuo A, Silverberg N, Fernandez Faith E, et al. A systematic scoping review of racial, ethnic, and socioeconomic health disparities in pediatric dermatology. Pediatr Dermatol 2021;38(Suppl 2):6–12. Epub 2021 Aug 18. PMID: 34409633.

20. Schmid-Grendelmeier P, Takaoka R, Ahogo KC, et al. Position Statement on Atopic Dermatitis in Sub-Saharan Africa: current status and roadmap. J Eur Acad Dermatol Venereol 2019;33(11): 2019–28. PMID: 31713914; PMCID: PMC6899619.

21. Silverberg N.B., Erythema in Children of Color. AAD Skin of Color Curriculum. Available at: https:// learning.aad.org/Listing/Skin-of-Color-Curriculum-5719. Accessed June 12, 2024.

22. Silverberg NB. Typical and atypical clinical appearance of atopic dermatitis. Clin Dermatol 2017; 35(4):354–9. Epub 2017 Mar 24. PMID: 28709565.

23. Rahma A, Lane ME. Skin Barrier Function in Infants: Update and Outlook. Pharmaceutics 2022;14(2): 433. PMID: 35214165; PMCID: PMC8880311.

24. Cury Martins J, Martins C, Aoki V, et al. Topical tacrolimus for atopic dermatitis. Cochrane Database Syst Rev 2015;2015(7):CD009864. PMID: 26132597; PMCID: PMC6461158.

25. Yu SH, Drucker AM, Lebwohl M, et al. A systematic review of the safety and efficacy of systemic corticosteroids in atopic dermatitis. J Am Acad Dermatol 2018;78(4):733–40.e11. Epub 2017 Dec 6. PMID: 29032119.

26. Silverberg JI, Garg NK, Paller AS, et al. Sleep disturbances in adults with eczema are associated with impaired overall health: a US population-based study. J Invest Dermatol 2015;135(1):56–66. Epub 2014 Aug 31. PMID: 25078665.

27. Silverberg JI, Paller AS. Association between eczema and stature in 9 US population-based studies. JAMA Dermatol 2015;151(4):401–9. PMID: 25493447.

28. Engel-Yeger B, Habib-Mazawi S, Parush S, et al. The sensory profile of children with atopic dermatitis as determined by the sensory profile questionnaire. J Am Acad Dermatol 2007;57(4):610–5. Epub 2007 Jun 18. PMID: 17574298.

29. Field T. Massage therapy for skin conditions in young children. Dermatol Clin 2005;23(4):717–21. PMID: 16112449.

30. Schachner L, Field T, Hernandez-Reif M, et al. Atopic dermatitis symptoms decreased in children following massage therapy. Pediatr Dermatol 1998; 15(5):390–5. PMID: 979659.

31. Lin L, Yu L, Zhang S, et al. The positive effect of mother-performed infant massage on infantile eczema and maternal mental state: A randomized controlled trial. Front Public Health 2023;10:1068043. https://doi.org/ 10.3389/fpubh.2022.1068043. PMID: 36711419; PMCID: PMC9875301.

32. Vernon HJ, Lane AT, Weston W. Comparison of mometasone furoate 0.1% cream and hydrocortisone 1.0% cream in the treatment of childhood atopic dermatitis. J Am Acad Dermatol 1991;24(4):603–7.

33. Chu DK, Chu AWL, Rayner DG, et al. Topical treatments for atopic dermatitis (eczema): Systematic review and network meta-analysis of randomized trials. J Allergy Clin Immunol 2023;152(6):1493–519. Epub 2023 Sep 9. PMID: 37678572.

34. Fonacier L, Banta E, Mawhirt S, et al. Capturing total steroid burden in patients with atopic dermatitis and asthma. Allergy Asthma Proc 2022;43(5):454–60. PMID: 36065113.

35. Brunner PM, Khattri S, Garcet S, et al. A mild topical steroid leads to progressive anti-inflammatory effects in the skin of patients with moderate-to-severe atopic dermatitis. J Allergy Clin Immunol 2016;138(1): 169–78. Epub 2016 Mar 2. PMID: 26948076.

36. Luger T, Chu CY, Elgendy A, et al. Pimecrolimus 1% cream for mild-to-moderate atopic dermatitis: a systematic review and meta-analysis with a focus on children and sensitive skin areas. Eur J Dermatol 2023;33(5):474–86. PMID: 38297923.

37. Geba GP, Li D, Xu M, et al. Attenuating the atopic march: Meta-analysis of the dupilumab atopic dermatitis database for incident allergic events. J Allergy Clin Immunol 2023;151(3):756–66. Epub 2022 Sep 7. PMID: 36084766.

38. Papp KA, Breuer K, Meurer M, et al. Long-term treatment of atopic dermatitis with pimecrolimus cream 1% in infants does not interfere with the development of protective antibodies after vaccination. J Am Acad Dermatol 2005;52(2):247–53. PMID: 15692469.

39. Blauvelt A, Simpson EL, Tyring SK, et al. Dupilumab does not affect correlates of vaccine-induced immunity: A randomized, placebo-controlled trial in adults with moderate-to-severe atopic dermatitis. J Am Acad Dermatol 2019;80(1):158–67.e1. Epub 2018 Aug 6. PMID: 30092324.

40. Martinez-Cabriales SA, Kirchhof MG, Constantinescu CM, et al. Recommendations for Vaccination in Children with Atopic Dermatitis Treated with Dupilumab: A Consensus Meeting, 2020. Am J Clin Dermatol 2021;22(4):443–55. Epub 2021 Jun 2. PMID: 34076879; PMCID: PMC8169786.

41. Siegfried EC, Wine Lee L, Spergel JM, et al. A case series of live attenuated vaccine administration in dupilumab-treated children with atopic dermatitis. Pediatr Dermatol 2024;41(2):204–9. Epub 2024 Feb 2. PMID: 38308453.

42. Eichenfield LF, Kusari A, Han AM, et al. Therapeutic education in atopic dermatitis: A position paper from the International Eczema Council. JAAD Int 2021;3: 8–13. PMID: 34409365; PMCID: PMC8361897.

43. Levy ML. Developing an eczema action plan. Clin Dermatol 2018;36(5):659–61. Epub 2018 Jun 8. PMID: 30217279.

44. Grossman SK, Schut C, Kupfer J, et al. Experiences with the first eczema school in the United States. Clin Dermatol 2018;36(5):662–7. Epub 2018 Jun 6. PMID: 30217280.

45. Paller AS, Siegfried EC, Cork MJ, et al. Infections in Children Aged 6 Months to 5 Years Treated with Dupilumab in a Placebo-Controlled Clinical Trial of Moderate-to-Severe Atopic Dermatitis. Paediatr Drugs 2024;26(2):163–73. Epub 2024 Jan 24. PMID: 38267692; PMCID: PMC10890978.

46. Gonzalez ME, Schaffer JV, Orlow SJ, et al. Cutaneous microbiome effects of fluticasone propionate cream and adjunctive bleach baths in childhood atopic dermatitis. J Am Acad Dermatol 2016;75(3): 481–93.e8. PMID: 27543211; PMCID: PMC4992571.

47. Huang JT, Abrams M, Tlougan B, et al. Treatment of Staphylococcus aureus colonization in atopic dermatitis decreases disease severity. Pediatrics 2009;123(5):e808–14. PMID: 19403473.

48. Moreau M, Seité S, Aguilar L, et al. aureus - Targeting Endolysin Significantly Improves Symptoms and QoL in Individuals With Atopic Dermatitis. J Drugs Dermatol 2021;20(12):1323–8. PMID: 34898160.

49. Roduit C, Frei R, Depner M, et al, The PASTURE study group. Phenotypes of Atopic Dermatitis Depending on the Timing of Onset and Progression in Childhood. JAMA Pediatr 2017;171(7):655–62. PMID: 28531273; PMCID: PMC5710337.

50. Roduit C, Frei R, Loss G, et al. Protection Against Allergy–Study in Rural Environments study group. Development of atopic dermatitis according to age of onset and association with early-life exposures. J Allergy Clin Immunol 2012;130(1):130–6.e5.

51. Roduit C, Frei R, Depner M, et al. PASTURE study group. Increased food diversity in the first year of life is inversely associated with allergic diseases. J Allergy Clin Immunol 2014;133(4):1056–64.

52. Müller S, Marenholz I, Lee YA, et al. Association of Filaggrin loss-of-function-mutations with atopic dermatitis and asthma in the Early Treatment of the Atopic Child (ETAC) population. Pediatr Allergy Immunol 2009;20(4):358–61. PMID: 19538357.

53. Allergic factors associated with the development of asthma and the influence of cetirizine in a double-blind, randomised, placebo-controlled trial: first results of ETAC. Early Treatment of the Atopic Child. Pediatr Allergy Immunol 1998;9(3):116–24. PMID: 9814724.

54. Warner JO. ETAC Study Group. Early Treatment of the Atopic Child. A double-blinded, randomized, placebo-controlled trial of cetirizine in preventing the onset of asthma in children with atopic dermatitis: 18 months' treatment and 18 months' posttreatment follow-up. J Allergy Clin Immunol 2001;108(6): 929–37. PMID: 11742270.

Management of Atopic Hand Dermatitis

Lauren R. Port, BA, Patrick M. Brunner, MD, MSc*

KEYWORDS

- Atopic hand dermatitis • Atopic hand eczema • Atopic dermatitis • Chronic hand eczema

KEY POINTS

- Atopic hand dermatitis is a debilitating skin disease that tends to take a chronic course and is often resistant to conventional treatments.
- A clear history and the identification of potential irritants and allergens are paramount for correct diagnosis and differentiation from other forms of chronic hand eczema.
- In recent years, a better insight into the pathophysiology of atopic dermatitis has helped to develop novel treatment approaches also for atopic hand dermatitis.
- Similar to atopic dermatitis, the treatment of atopic hand dermatitis follows a stepwise approach from topical to systemic therapeutics.

INTRODUCTION

Atopic dermatitis (AD), also known as atopic eczema, is a chronic inflammatory skin disease that is characterized by highly pruritic lesions, commonly triggered by environmental irritants and allergens.[1] Atopic hand dermatitis (AHD) is a specific manifestation of AD in which the aforementioned symptoms are found primarily on the back of the hands, the inner wrists, and the base of the fingers.[2] AHD is considered a multifactorial disease with a complex etiopathogenesis, with genetic predisposition being a major risk factor, but epigenetic modifications and environmental exposures likely also play a key role in its development.[3] Further risk factors include age, pregnancy, geographic location, and environmental exposure,[4] but the exact pathogenesis is still only incompletely understood.

PATHOGENESIS

The pathogenesis of AD most likely involves a combination of many factors, including genetic predisposition, exacerbated immune responses, skin and gut microbiome changes, a compromised skin barrier, and environmental triggers.[5,6] A complex combination of inflammatory cells, cytokines, and chemokines is involved in its pathogenesis, resulting particularly in dysregulated Th2, but also Th22 and Th9 immune axes.[6,7] Loss of function mutations in the filaggrin gene are notable for their strong association with AD development.[8] With a loss of integrity to the epidermal barrier, irritants, allergens, and other pathogens can more easily invade the skin, which then mounts a pathologic immune response.[9]

Besides filaggrin, tight junctions play an important role in the defense system of the skin barrier and reduced expression of the claudin-1 protein, for instance, causes skin barrier disruption in AD.[10] Moreover, AD is characterized by insufficient upregulation of antimicrobial peptides due to strong Th2 activation.[11] This combined lack of defense mechanisms increases susceptibility to secondary colonization of organisms like *Staphylococcus aureus*.[11]

Similar to AD, AHD also can arise due to a combination of genetic factors and environmental triggers. Within the broad category of environmental exposures, AHD can be specifically triggered by

Department of Dermatology, Icahn School of Medicine at Mount Sinai, One Gustave L Levy Place, New York, NY 10029, USA
* Corresponding author.
E-mail address: patrick.brunner@mountsinai.org

Dermatol Clin 42 (2024) 619–623
https://doi.org/10.1016/j.det.2024.06.002

work environments across various professions, especially those that require the hands to have frequent contact with irritants and allergens.[12] Health care workers, hairdressers, food industry workers, plumbers, and mechanics are some examples.[13] Among nurses, for instance, frequent handwashing has been specifically identified as the primary precipitant of AHD.[14] In this regard, however, it is essential to distinguish between AHD and related conditions such as contact dermatitis, both irritant (ICD) and allergic (ACD).[15] ICD is a response to direct exposure of an irritant to the skin and a resulting inflammatory response, hypothesized to involve activation of the innate immune system. By contrast, ACD is classified as a type IV hypersensitivity response by the adaptive immune system, namely antigen-specific T lymphocytes.[16] For both ACD and ICD, AD is an important risk factor but does not completely explain their development.[17] Compared to both types of contact dermatitis, the pathogenesis behind AHD is generally believed to result from a more complex interaction between genetic predispositions, environmental exposures, and immune pathways.[18]

BURDEN OF DISEASE

Living with a condition as visible as AHD can bring immense physical and emotional discomfort into the patient's everyday life.[19] The unpredictable fluctuation of symptoms and the visibility of AHD can have a profound negative impact on health-related quality of life. AHD can compromise an individual's capacity to execute tasks properly in their workplace or even attend work at all.[20,21] This convergence of physical discomfort and disease visibility helps to emphasize the importance of a correct diagnosis to choose an efficacious treatment modality.

DIAGNOSIS

AD itself is typically a clinical diagnosis. Complementary tests include skin swabs, patch testing, serum IgE measurements, and skin prick or scratch testing.[22] In contrast to other chronic inflammatory conditions, a skin biopsy is not generally beneficial, as histology cannot differentiate between different etiologies of chronic hand eczema.[23–25] Importantly, different ages have shown their unique lesion distribution.[26] While the severity of the disease is usually assessed clinically, some biomarkers can also be used such as serum LDH and CCL17, which are generally increased in patients with moderate-to-severe AD.[27] For AHD, a patient's past medical history plays an important role in the differentiation between AHD and ICD or

ACD. Importantly, patients with AD have higher frequencies of allergies than the general population. On average, 50% of children and 35% of adults suffering from AD are sensitized to common allergens.[28–31] Similarly, chronic hand eczema patients have an increased risk of allergic sensitization, and top ACD allergens haven been shown to include nickel, fragrances, quaternium-15, benzalkonium chloride, and methylisothiazolinone.[32–34] Thus, patch testing is an important diagnostic tool for the differentiation of ICD from ACD.

MANAGEMENT AND TREATMENT

Due to a better understanding of AD pathogenesis, there has been a revolution in treatment options for AHD, particularly due to the advent of biologics and small molecules that have recently become available.[35] Nevertheless, patient counseling about proper skin care practices and topical treatment modalities including moisturizers, corticosteroids, and calcineurin inhibitors are particularly important aspects of the treatment plan for AHD patients.[36]

Similar to AD, the approach for AHD treatment is directly proportional to the severity of the condition. Topical corticosteroids and calcineurin inhibitors are generally prescribed first, followed by higher potency topical corticosteroids and UV therapy, and, if not sufficient, systemic therapeutic modalities.[37] Wet wrap therapy has long been used to boost the efficacy of topical treatments and is still an important treatment strategy.[38] Calcipotriol, a derivative of vitamin D3, has efficacy for chronic hand eczema patients.[39] Crisaborole, a PDE-4 inhibitor, has been approved for patients with AD and can also improve AHD symptoms.[40,41]

The topical application of JAK inhibitors is currently being investigated in several trials for chronic hand eczema. Delgocitinib is a pan-JAK inhibitor that has shown overall improvement in hand eczema,[42] and ruxolitinib, a JAK1 and JAK2 inhibitor, also showed positive data for its improvement of pruritic symptoms in hand eczema patients, and has been approved for the treatment of AD.[39,43,44] Importantly, these topical treatments have only been investigated short term, and their long-term safety still needs to be established.

Regarding the use of phototherapy, psoralen and ultraviolet A (PUVA) and narrow-band ultraviolet B (NB-UVB) have been proven to reduce symptoms of AHD. Using a 308 nm excimer laser is another treatment option for chronic hand eczema that could potentially serve as a replacement for other UV therapies due to its ability to target smaller areas at a lower dose of UV radiation.[45]

There are now several recently approved systemic therapies available for AD. IL-4 and/or IL-13 inhibitors (dupilumab, tralokinumab, and lebrikizumab) target type 2 inflammatory immune pathways.[46,47] JAK inhibitors (abrocitinib, upadacitinib, and baricitinib) have also proven effective treatments for AD, which more broadly target cytokine pathways.[42] While most of these agents are approved for the treatment of moderate-to-severe AD, their impact specifically on AHD is less clear.

Dupilumab has specifically demonstrated positive results in trials for AD patients with chronic hand eczema.[48,49] While tralokinumab and lebrikizumab showed improved symptoms and overall quality of life for patients with AD, their impact on hand manifestations has not been analyzed as robustly as dupilumab.[42,46,50] Alitretinoin is a vitamin A derivative and has been approved in various countries for chronic hand eczema. It works by targeting retinoic acid receptors, improving symptoms of inflammation. However, there are side effects that arise after prolonged use, including but not limited to headaches, teratogenicity, alopecia, and myalgias.[39,51] Systemic immunosuppressants such as cyclosporine, azathioprine, methotrexate, and mycophenolate mofetil have also been explored as a possible treatment option for patients with chronic hand eczema.[37] However, these oral immunosuppressants can have a wide range of adverse effects and patient monitoring is necessary.[2,39]

As for systemic JAK inhibitors, there has been recent research addressing their treatment specifically for hand eczema patients, particularly with atopic predispositions.[42,43] Gusacitinib has been shown to suppress the underlying inflammatory response in patients with hand eczema.[52] Baricitinib is another systemic JAK inhibitor that has displayed improvement for patients with AD but has not been profoundly researched for patients with hand eczema specifically,[43] but a case series showed improvement in patients with chronic hand eczema.[53] Upadacitinib, a small molecule JAK inhibitor, has exhibited positive signs of improvement in the treatment of AD patients with atopic hand eczema in 2 randomized phase-3 trials.[54] Abrocitinib has also been approved for the treatment of moderate-to-severe AD and showed efficacy for AHD.[55] Overall, the rapidly increasing group of JAK inhibitors show promising results for various forms of eczema; however, their efficacy will need to be weighted in light of their long-term safety data, which are often not yet available.

SUMMARY

Recent developments in AD treatment also have a profound impact on treatment modalities of AHD.

While many patients can now be treated with better efficacy, more research is still needed to identify optimal care for the patient with AHD.

CLINICS CARE POINTS

- AHD can be a debilitating skin disease, that needs to be distinguished from allergic and irritant contact dermatitis.
- Novel treatment approaches are currently revolutionizing the care of patients with AD, including those with AHD.

DISCLOSURES

P.M. Brunner has received personal fees from Almirall, Sanofi, Janssen, LEO Pharma, AbbVie, Pfizer, Boehringer Ingelheim, GSK, Regeneron, Eli Lilly, Celgene, Novartis, UCB, Merck, RAPT Therapeutics, Galderma, and BMS. P.M. Brunner has received research support from Pfizer, United States (grant paid to his institution). L.R. Port declares no relevant conflicts of interest.

REFERENCES

1. Silverberg JI, Simpson B, Abuabara K, et al. Prevalence and burden of atopic dermatitis involving the head, neck, face, and hand: A cross sectional study from the TARGET-DERM AD cohort. J Am Acad Dermatol 2023;89(3):519–28.

2. Chan CX, Zug KA. Diagnosis and Management of Dermatitis, Including Atopic, Contact, and Hand Eczemas. Med Clin North Am 2021;105(4):611–26.

3. Nutten S. Atopic dermatitis: global epidemiology and risk factors. Ann Nutr Metab 2015;66(Suppl 1):8–16.

4. Kantor R, Silverberg JI. Environmental risk factors and their role in the management of atopic dermatitis. Expet Rev Clin Immunol 2017;13(1):15–26.

5. Schuler CF, Billi AC, Maverakis E, et al. Novel insights into atopic dermatitis. J Allergy Clin Immunol 2023;151(5):1145–54.

6. Rothenberg-Lausell C, Bar J, Del Duca E, et al. Diversity of atopic dermatitis and selection of immune targets. Ann Allergy Asthma Immunol 2023. https://doi.org/10.1016/j.anai.2023.11.020.

7. Li H, Zhang Z, Zhang H, et al. Update on the Pathogenesis and Therapy of Atopic Dermatitis. Clin Rev Allergy Immunol 2021;61(3):324–38.

8. Stefanovic N, Irvine AD. Filaggrin and beyond: New insights into the skin barrier in atopic dermatitis and allergic diseases, from genetics to therapeutic perspectives. Ann Allergy Asthma Immunol 2024;132(2):187–95.

9. Peng W, Novak N. Pathogenesis of atopic dermatitis. Clin Exp Allergy 2015;45(3):566–74.

10. Beck LA, Cork MJ, Amagai M, et al. Type 2 Inflammation Contributes to Skin Barrier Dysfunction in Atopic Dermatitis. JID Innov 2022;2(5):100131.

11. Nakatsuji T, Chen TH, Narala S, et al. Antimicrobials from human skin commensal bacteria protect against Staphylococcus aureus and are deficient in atopic dermatitis. Sci Transl Med 2017;9(378). https://doi.org/10.1126/scitranslmed.aah4680.

12. Ruff SMD, Engebretsen KA, Zachariae C, et al. The association between atopic dermatitis and hand eczema: a systematic review and meta-analysis. Br J Dermatol 2018;178(4):879–88.

13. Lampel HP, Powell HB. Occupational and Hand Dermatitis: a Practical Approach. Clin Rev Allergy Immunol 2019;56(1):60–71.

14. Hui-Beckman J, Leung DYM, Goleva E. Hand hygiene impact on the skin barrier in health care workers and individuals with atopic dermatitis. Ann Allergy Asthma Immunol 2022;128(1):108–10.

15. Loman L, Brands MJ, Massella Patsea AAL, et al. Lifestyle factors and hand eczema: A systematic review and meta-analysis of observational studies. Contact Dermatitis 2022;87(3):211–32.

16. Tancredi V, Buononato D, Caccavale S, et al. New perspectives in the management of chronic hand eczema: lessons from pathogenesis. Int J Mol Sci 2023;25(1). https://doi.org/10.3390/ijms25010362.

17. Lerbaek A, Kyvik KO, Mortensen J, et al. Heritability of hand eczema is not explained by comorbidity with atopic dermatitis. J Invest Dermatol 2007;127(7):1632–40.

18. Thyssen JP, Johansen JD, Linneberg A, et al. The epidemiology of hand eczema in the general population–prevalence and main findings. Contact Dermatitis 2010;62(2):75–87.

19. Barrett A, Hahn-Pedersen J, Kragh N, et al. Patient-reported outcome measures in atopic dermatitis and chronic hand eczema in adults. Patient 2019;12(5):445–59.

20. Capucci S, Hahn-Pedersen J, Vilsboll A, et al. Impact of atopic dermatitis and chronic hand eczema on quality of life compared with other chronic diseases. Dermatitis May/2020;31(3):178–84.

21. Chen YC, Wu CS, Lu YW, et al. Atopic dermatitis and non-atopic hand eczema have similar negative impacts on quality of life: implications for clinical significance. Acta Derm Venereol 2013;93(6):749–50.

22. Weidinger S, Beck LA, Bieber T, et al. Atopic dermatitis. Nat Rev Dis Primers 2018;4(1):1.

23. Vestergaard L, Clemmensen OJ, Sorensen FB, et al. Histological distinction between early allergic and irritant patch test reactions: follicular spongiosis may be characteristic of early allergic contact dermatitis. Contact Dermatitis 1999;41(4):207–10.

24. Frings VG, Boer-Auer A, Breuer K. Histomorphology and Immunophenotype of Eczematous Skin Lesions Revisited-Skin Biopsies Are Not Reliable in Differentiating Allergic Contact Dermatitis, Irritant Contact Dermatitis, and Atopic Dermatitis. Am J Dermatopathol 2018;40(1):7–16.

25. Silverberg JI, Guttman-Yassky E, Agner T, et al. Chronic Hand Eczema Guidelines From an Expert Panel of the International Eczema Council. Dermatitis 2021;32(5):319–26.

26. Napolitano M, Fabbrocini G, Martora F, et al. Children atopic dermatitis: Diagnosis, mimics, overlaps, and therapeutic implication. Dermatol Ther 2022;35(12):e15901.

27. Kou K, Aihara M, Matsunaga T, et al. Association of serum interleukin-18 and other biomarkers with disease severity in adults with atopic dermatitis. Arch Dermatol Res 2012;304(4):305–12.

28. Schafer T. The impact of allergy on atopic eczema from data from epidemiological studies. Curr Opin Allergy Clin Immunol 2008;8(5):418–22.

29. Schafer T, Kramer U, Vieluf D, et al. The excess of atopic eczema in East Germany is related to the intrinsic type. Br J Dermatol 2000;143(5):992–8.

30. Flohr C, Johansson SG, Wahlgren CF, et al. How atopic is atopic dermatitis? J Allergy Clin Immunol 2004;114(1):150–8.

31. Eller E, Kjaer HF, Host A, et al. Food allergy and food sensitization in early childhood: results from the DARC cohort. Allergy 2009;64(7):1023–9.

32. Silverberg JI, Patel N, Warshaw EM, et al. Hand and foot dermatitis in patients referred for patch testing: Analysis of North American Contact Dermatitis Group Data, 2001-2018. J Am Acad Dermatol 2022;87(5):1049–59.

33. Agner T, Aalto-Korte K, Andersen KE, et al. Factors associated with combined hand and foot eczema. J Eur Acad Dermatol Venereol 2017;31(5):828–32.

34. Lopez-Castillo D, Descalzo MA, Olmos-Alpiste F, et al. Chronic hand eczema: clinical characterization, aetiology, concomitant foot eczema and poly-sensitization. Eur J Dermatol 2022;32(1):99–106.

35. Czarnowicki T, He H, Krueger JG, et al. Atopic dermatitis endotypes and implications for targeted therapeutics. J Allergy Clin Immunol 2019;143(1):1–11.

36. Halling-Overgaard AS, Zachariae C, Thyssen JP. Management of Atopic Hand Dermatitis. Dermatol Clin 2017;35(3):365–72.

37. Antonov D, Schliemann S, Elsner P. Hand dermatitis: a review of clinical features, prevention and treatment. Am J Clin Dermatol 2015;16(4):257–70.

38. Nicol NH, Boguniewicz M. Wet Wrap Therapy in Moderate to Severe Atopic Dermatitis. Immunol Allergy Clin North Am 2017;37(1):123–39.

39. Dubin C, Del Duca E, Guttman-Yassky E. Drugs for the Treatment of Chronic Hand Eczema: Successes

and Key Challenges. Ther Clin Risk Manag 2020;16:1319–32.

40. Cheng J, Facheris P, Ungar B, et al. Current emerging and investigational drugs for the treatment of chronic hand eczema. Expert Opin Investig Drugs 2022;31(8):843–53.

41. Kahn JS, Grossman-Kranseler JS, Zancanaro P, et al. Topical Crisaborole in the Treatment of Atopic Hand Dermatitis: A Retrospective Chart Review. Dermatitis 2021;32(6):e141–3.

42. Ho JSS, Molin S. A Review of Existing and New Treatments for the Management of Hand Eczema. J Cutan Med Surg 2023;27(5):493–503.

43. Zalewski A, Szepietowski JC. Topical and systemic JAK inhibitors in hand eczema - a narrative review. Expet Rev Clin Immunol 2023;19(4):365–73.

44. Worm M, Thyssen JP, Schliemann S, et al. The pan-JAK inhibitor delgocitinib in a cream formulation demonstrates dose response in chronic hand eczema in a 16-week randomized phase IIb trial. Br J Dermatol 2022;187(1):42–51.

45. Shroff A, Malajian D, Czarnowicki T, et al. Use of 308 nm excimer laser for the treatment of chronic hand and foot eczema. Int J Dermatol 2016;55(8):e447–53.

46. Dubin C, Del Duca E, Guttman-Yassky E. The IL-4, IL-13 and IL-31 pathways in atopic dermatitis. Expert Rev Clin Immunol 2021;17(8):835–52.

47. Simpson EL, Bieber T, Guttman-Yassky E, et al. Two Phase 3 Trials of Dupilumab versus Placebo in Atopic Dermatitis. N Engl J Med 2016;375(24):2335–48.

48. Oosterhaven JAF, Voorberg AN, Romeijn GLE, et al. Effect of dupilumab on hand eczema in patients with atopic dermatitis: An observational study. J Dermatol 2019;46(8):680–5.

49. Simpson EL, Silverberg JI, Worm M, et al. Dupilumab treatment improves signs, symptoms, quality of life, and work productivity in patients with atopic hand and foot dermatitis: Results from a phase 3, randomized, double-blind, placebo-controlled trial. J Am Acad Dermatol 2024;90(6):1190–9.

50. Singh R, Taylor A, Shah MA, et al. Review of Tralokinumab in the Treatment of Atopic Dermatitis. Ann Pharmacother 2023;57(3):333–40.

51. Seol JE, Kim JU, Hong SM, et al. Alitretinoin Compliance in Patients with Chronic Hand Eczema. Ann Dermatol 2021;33(1):46–51.

52. Jimenez PA, Sofen HL, Bissonnette R, et al. Oral spleen tyrosine kinase/Janus Kinase inhibitor gusacitinib for the treatment of chronic hand eczema: Results of a randomized phase 2 study. J Am Acad Dermatol 2023;89(2):235–42.

53. Lee SD, Ahn HJ, Shin MK. Nine cases of chronic hand and foot eczema treated with baricitinib. Australas J Dermatol 2023;64(3):408–12.

54. Simpson EL, Rahawi K, Hu X, et al. Effect of upadacitinib on atopic hand eczema in patients with moderate-to-severe atopic dermatitis: Results from two randomized phase 3 trials. J Eur Acad Dermatol Venereol 2023;37(9):1863–70.

55. Kamphuis E, Boesjes CM, Loman L, et al. Real-world Experience of Abrocitinib Treatment in Patients with Atopic Dermatitis and Hand Eczema: Up to 28-week Results from the BioDay Registry. Acta Derm Venereol 2024;104:adv19454.

Exploring the Association Between Atopic Dermatitis and Malignancy

A Comprehensive Review with Therapeutic Strategies

David L. Drum, BS[a], Leo S. Wan, BA[b], Anika G. Jallorina, BS[a], Mary F. Lee-Wong, MD, MS, MSc[c],*

KEYWORDS

• Eczema • Pruritus • Cancer • Atopic dermatitis treatment • Malignancies

KEY POINTS

• Atopic dermatitis (AD) is a chronic disease of the skin characterized by itchy papules and patches located on the body's flexor surfaces.
• It is caused by a Th2 response to enhanced antigen exposure due to an impaired skin barrier. There is speculation that this increased immune response could offer protective effects or elevate the risk of certain cancers.
• Skin cancers, such as basal cell carcinoma (BCC) and squamous cell carcinoma (SCC), were found to have an increased association with AD, with several risk factors being considered. One important confounder is patients with AD were more likely to be seen by a dermatologist.
• Inflammation may extend beyond the skin to the gastrointestinal system, brain, and lungs where increased immune response seems to explain why AD has mostly inverse associations with cancers. Whereas, in hematologic malignancies, chronic inflammation may increase susceptibility to various types of disease.

INTRODUCTION

Atopic dermatitis (AD) is a dermatologic condition that affects 20% of children and 10% of adults and can present as dry, scaly, pruritic papules, patches, and plaques. Onset is usually before the age of 5.

Previously, the etiology of AD was commonly attributed to either a compromised skin epidermal barrier, resulting in heightened exposure to antigens that trigger an immune response, or dysregulation within the immune system. However, a more comprehensive model has emerged, combining elements of both theories. In this model, overactivation of immune components due to increased exposure to antigens ultimately leads to a cascade of immune responses orchestrated by Th2 and Th17 cells.[1] Recent focus has been on neuroimmunology, the skin microbiome, and lipid content.[2] The immunologic reaction leads to an impaired skin barrier with dermal mast cell invasion and clinical features, such as spongiosis, acanthosis, and hyperkeratosis, usually with accumulation of Th2 cells.[3] The damaged skin barrier, as well as the heightened immunologic response in AD, may suggest conflicting correlations with

[a] California University of Science and Medicine, Colton, CA 92324, USA; [b] West Virginia School of Osteopathic Medicine, Lewisburg, WV 24901, USA; [c] Department of Medicine, Division of Allergy and Immunology, Icahn School of Medicine at Mount Sinai, New York, NY 10019, USA
* Corresponding author.
E-mail address: MLWong@maimonidesmed.org

Dermatol Clin 42 (2024) 625–634
https://doi.org/10.1016/j.det.2024.06.001

derm.theclinics.com

malignancies. It is unclear whether the impaired epidermal barrier may increase susceptibility of certain malignancies or whether the exaggerated immune system may decrease cancer susceptibility. Thus, the correlation between AD and malignancy may vary by cancer type.

One significant factor contributing to the conflicting results in studies analyzing the association of AD and cancer is the variability in study design. Some studies rely on patient self-reporting to establish the study population, while others utilize hospital discharge information. Importantly, studies usually do not account for other factors known to influence cancer risk, such as smoking history, family history, and occupation exposure. Differences in cancer rates across various countries complicate cross-study comparison. Variations in sun exposure, diet, and genetics also significantly impact the development of malignancy.[4]

The authors explore the implications of AD's pathogenesis for skin cancers, solid tumors, and hematologic malignancies. Chronic inflammation associated with AD induces alterations in the immune system, potentially increasing the risk of developing various hematologic malignancies in the future.

PROPOSED MECHANISMS OF ATOPIC DERMATITIS ASSOCIATION WITH MALIGNANCY

Some have proposed that AD serves a protective role against the formation of malignancy due to constant activation of the immune system, allowing for early detection of tumor neoantigens and leading to the prompt removal by the immune system before the cancer can progress. Others suggest it may create an inflammatory state that is damaging to normal cells with the increased cell turnover creating an environment that is susceptible to cancer formation.[5]

In addition, the authors delved into how treatments for AD can influence its association with malignancy. With the emergence of new biologic agents targeting complex molecular pathways such as JAK-STAT, IL-4, and IL-13, the authors examined the associations of these pathways with specific cancers. This exploration laid the groundwork for questioning how inhibition of these pathways may affect the association of AD with cancers in the future. By understanding the intricate connections between these treatment targets and cancer pathways, the authors could better anticipate the potential impacts of novel AD therapies on risk of malignancy.

SKIN MALIGNANCIES
Melanoma

The link between melanoma and AD was extensively studied by physicians and scientists. Nielsen and colleagues developed and described a competitive ELISA approach that targets the N-terminal of COL6-α6-chain in type VI collagen, known as C6A6. Their objective was to evaluate C6A6's association, relative to healthy controls, with a number of dermatologic disorders, such as cutaneous malignant melanoma, hidradenitis suppurativa, urticaria, vitiligo, systemic lupus erythematosus, AD, and psoriasis.[6] C6A6 levels were shown to be significantly higher in patients with both AD and melanoma, indicating a possible relationship between the two conditions.[6]

In another study by Nguyen and colleagues, the group examined tissue samples from various skin disorders, such as melanomas and AD, using immunohistochemical techniques to investigate the expression of integrins β6 and β8.[7] Although high expression of integrin β6 was extensively established across numerous cancer types, the significance of integrin β8 remains unclear. According to recent studies, tumor cells that express β8 may be able to activate TGFβ, which will subsequently promote the differentiation and enrichment of regulatory T cells and ultimately accelerate the growth of tumors.[7] Interestingly, integrin β6 expression was found to be elevated in AD samples, although integrin β8 levels stayed unchanged. Contrastingly, integrin β6 was not expressed in most melanomas, which exhibited significant amounts of integrin β8.[7]

Eight separate studies exploring the connection between melanoma risk and AD were examined in a meta-analysis by Gandini and colleagues. Of these, four were case-control studies while the other four were large cohort studies.[8] The results of these investigations, however, paint a somewhat contradictory picture. This discrepancy is mostly due to the fact that the research designs and study subjects' characteristics vary widely between the studies. Cohort studies have the benefit of potentially quantifying the latency between AD and melanoma since they follow AD patients from the time of hospital discharge onwards. However, they frequently fall short of accounting for potential confounding variables, such as UVB exposure and phenotypic characteristics. Conversely, case-control studies may be able to overcome these drawbacks. However, they are more prone to exposure misclassification. This is partly because the diagnosis of AD may have occurred a long time ago and is often self-reported, introducing the possibility of recall bias into the study.[8]

Also, research has explored the possible relationship between melanoma risk and AD treatment options. Lam and colleagues conducted a systematic review and meta-analysis to investigate the relationship between topical calcineurin inhibitors (TCIs) and the risk of several malignancies, including lymphoma, keratinocyte carcinoma, and melanoma. TCIs are often used as a second-line treatment for AD; however, because of their immunosuppressive effects, the United States Food and Drug Administration (FDA) have issued a black box warning about the possibility of malignancy.[9]

In this study, separate analyses were performed for cohort and case-control studies, with the meta-analysis limited to cohort studies. The researchers discovered that using TCIs did not increase the likelihood of developing melanoma, despite worries about their immunosuppressive qualities.[9]

Basal Cell Carcinoma

In the United States, basal cell carcinoma (BCC) is the most frequent skin cancer.[10] The Veterans Affairs Topical Tretinoin Chemoprevention Trial, developed by Dyer and colleagues, was a noteworthy study that examined predictors of new BCCs in a high-risk population. The study included 1131 participants, with 97% being male and 57% having pursued higher education to some extent. The average age of participants in this group was 72 years, and all participants exhibited significant sun-damaged skin.[10] Almost 44% of the individuals experienced the onset of new BCC cases over an average follow-up period of 3.6 years. A comprehensive multivariate analysis model was created for this study. Initially, the model integrated all the risk factors associated with the development of new BCC at a P-value less than 0.15, using a stepwise backward regression approach. History of AD emerged as a singular risk factor for future BCC cases, with a hazard rate ratio of 1.52 (95% confidence interval of 1.01–2.29). It is notable that participants with AD, within this context, did not report using TCIs. Although, the determination of AD was based on self-reported diagnoses that were told by physicians.[10]

Additionally, another cohort investigation by Jensen and colleagues indicated an increased risk of BCC among patients diagnosed with both AD and asthma, showing a 41% greater likelihood of developing BCC (standardized incidence ratio [SIR] of 1.41; 95% confidence interval [CI] of 1.07 to 1.83). However, the presence of AD alone did not significantly elevate the risk for BCC (SIR of 1.29; 95% CI of 0.92–1.77), indicating a complex interplay of factors contributing to the risk of developing BCC.[11]

Researchers have long been interested in the association between AD and BCC, although substantial causation has yet to be shown. Studies on this subject may yield different results depending on a number of factors. First, because AD can cause persistent inflammation or require the use of immunosuppressive medications, it could increase the chance of developing BCC. Patients with AD may also have a higher diagnosis rate of BCC since they see dermatologists more frequently. As a result, individuals with AD may consequently have a higher reported incidence of BCC.[12]

Squamous Cell Carcinoma

Similar to the conflicting results concerning BCC and melanoma, the research on the relationship between squamous cell carcinoma (SCC) and AD is also unclear. Cho and colleagues conducted a retrospective, case-control analysis in which they identified 399 participants with a history of SCC that were documented and compared them with 780 controls who had no history of SCC in order to investigate this possible connection.[13] The confounding factors in this investigation, such as race, smoking history, ionizing radiation exposure, and use of immunosuppressants, were carefully considered.[13] With an adjusted odds ratio of 1.75 (95% CI, 1.05–2.93), the results showed a strong correlation between SCC and AD, supporting the findings of a few earlier studies.[11,14,15] However, it is vital to consider potential surveillance biases that may influence these results, patients with SCC are likely to seek dermatologic care more frequently than those without, and the increased prevalence of non-SCC cancers among patients with SCC could lead to heightened dermatologic surveillance.[16]

Furthermore, Zhu and colleagues performed a systematic review and qualitative analysis to investigate the link between AD and several types of skin cancer, including SCC. A review of three studies found that people with AD have a significantly increased risk of SCC (odds ratio [OR] 1.90, 95% CI 1.33–2.72, P_heterogeneity = 0.770, I^2 = 0.0%).[16] Notably, this study incorporated a confounding factor that has not been previously addressed: the frequent use of phototherapy in AD patients, which may contribute to an elevated risk of skin cancers. However, it is critical to acknowledge the potential limits of systematic studies, such as unavoidable high heterogeneity, variations in adjustment factors among studies, and a geographic bias favoring studies from Europe and North America. These limitations highlight the necessity for more diverse studies that include information from non-Western nations in order to offer a more comprehensive understanding of risks connected to AD.[16]

GASTROINTESTINAL MALIGNANCIES
Colorectal Cancer

Several studies found a decreased incidence of colorectal cancer (CRC) in patients with AD[17,18] suggesting a potential link between inflammation and enhanced immune surveillance within the intestinal mucosa. Also, inverse association with AD was found in a predominantly French population in Quebec when looking at 437 patients diagnosed with CRC (OR = 0.73).[19] Similarly, a register-based retrospective cohort study in Sweden, encompassing over 15000 AD hospitalized patients, observed a SIR of 0.7 for CRC development.[14]

Use of Mendelian randomization found a correlation with the TET2 gene, implicated in both AD and CRC. Reduced expression of TET2 was associated with worse outcomes in CRC and increased lymphatic metastasis. This shared gene is also associated with immune system response and regulation through pathways that control T cell and macrophage differentiation.[20]

Contrarily, a recent study in Taiwan surveying 138510 patients, 27702 of whom have AD, revealed an association between AD and CRC (HR = 1.26) across all age groups above the ages of 20, irrespective of gender. They also saw an increased association between the number of patient visits per year for AD and CRC.[21] Eight years previously using the same database in Taiwan, it had been reported by Hwang and colleagues that there was an inverse association of CRC with males (SIR = 0.83) and increased SIR with females (SIR = 1.24).[22] While the authors are hesitant to draw direct cross-study conclusions, dupilumab was approved in Taiwan during the time between the two studies, which brings a new dynamic to the immune response associated with AD.

In Europe, it was found that CRC was correlated with increased levels of IL-13.[23] While an overall consensus has not been reached on the association between AD, IL-13, and CRC, future research exploring the impact of IL-13-targeted therapies on this association will be crucial.

Esophageal Cancer

A Mendelian randomization study investigated the susceptibility of both East Asian and European populations to esophageal carcinoma in individuals diagnosed with AD. Esophageal carcinoma mostly occurs in the East Asian population and is heavily skewed toward esophageal SCC compared to adenocarcinoma.[24] This study found that there was a connection between AD and a reduced susceptibility to esophageal cancer in East Asians, but no correlation was found in Europeans.[25] Another study in Europe looking specifically at the Swedish population found an SIR of 3.5.[14] These findings suggest that genetic or environmental differences may influence the varying degrees of protection or lack thereof conferred by AD against esophageal cancer.

Interestingly, the impact of AD on esophageal cancer risk may also vary by gender, as evidenced by a study involving 295466 patients in Korea. Men exhibited an inverse association (HR = 0.85) while women have an increased association (HR = 1.46).[18]

When considering important cytokines in AD pathogenesis, IL-13 was detected in esophageal SCC via immunohistochemistry staining and correlated with a favorable prognosis. High IL-13 density at every TNM classification of esophageal SCC could predict low and high risk groups.[26] These findings suggest that AD may indeed confer protection against esophageal cancer in certain populations, with the key cytokine IL-13 playing a significant role in both the development of AD and the prognosis of esophageal cancer.

Stomach Cancer

In Korea, a study showed inverse association between AD and the development of stomach cancer (HR = 0.97) for both men and women.[18] Similarly, a case-control study in Montreal found an inverse association of AD and stomach cancer among 227 adults diagnosed with stomach cancer (OR = 0.5).[19]

However, contrasting results were found from a study in Sweden, where an increased SIR of 1.1 was observed for AD and stomach cancer among patients hospitalized for AD over a 35-year period.[14] It is worth noting that while this result contradicts the inverse association reported in previous studies, the Swedish study focused on patients hospitalized for AD, whereas the Montreal study relied on self-reported AD status among cancer patients. These differing approaches to the data collection may underscore the discrepancies in association and highlight one of the primary challenges in reaching a consensus regarding the risk of AD and stomach cancer.

HEMATOLOGICAL MALIGNANCIES
Acute Lymphoblastic Leukemia

A recent meta-analysis by Liang and colleagues that pooled data from studies conducted across America, Europe, and Asia (n = 7) found an inverse association (OR = 0.76) between AD and acute lymphoblastic leukemia (ALL). This reduced risk may be due to commonly used treatments for AD, such as glucocorticoids, that are also used in ALL.[27] Furthermore, recently FDA-approved therapies for AD like JAK inhibitors, such as upadacitinib and abrocitinib, which are potent JAK1 inhibitors,[28,29] may also have a protective effect against ALL. Upadacitinib and abrocitinib have similar rates of malignancy association showing that selection of one does not favor increased risk of developing cancer.[30]

The JAK-STAT pathway is composed of three main components. Cytokines like IL-4 and IL-13, pivotal in AD, bind to receptors on the cell surface, initiating phosphorylation of JAKs located on the cytoplasmic membrane. This phosphorylation enables STATs, via their SH2 domains, to bind and undergo phosphorylation. Subsequently, phosphorylated STATs translocate to the nucleus, causing changes in gene expression of pathways that affect immune cells function, proliferation, and maturation.[31]

Studies of B cell and T cell ALL found mutations in the IL-7 complex that includes JAK1 and JAK3.[32] To potentially combat this mechanism, JAK inhibitors are currently being evaluated in clinical trials for ALL.[33]

Hodgkin's Lymphoma

Liang and colleagues found that AD was associated with increased risk in Hodgkin's lymphoma (HL) (OR = 1.66) based on data from six studies in America and Europe.[27] Another meta-analysis looking at four cohort studies (relative risk [RR] = 1.43) and 18 case-control studies (OR = 1.18) reported AD and increased severity of AD were associated with increased risk of multiple types of lymphoma including HL.[34]

Notably, the IL-4/IL-13/STAT6/Bcl-xl axis, which is upregulated in HL to promote cell survival, was shown to induce apoptosis upon blockade.[35] Furthermore, JAK inhibitors demonstrated the ability to inhibit cellular proliferation in HL, potentially influencing future associations between AD and HL.[36]

Cutaneous T Cell Lymphomas

The association between AD and cutaneous T cell lymphoma (CTCL) is complex as the two conditions often present with similar symptoms, such as pruritic erythematous plaques, leading to confusion in diagnosis.[37] Both AD and CTCL involve dysregulation of Th2 cells, with CTCL exhibiting elevated levels of these T cells, along with increased immunoglobin (Ig) E and IgA in

serum. T cells in CTCL are phenotypically T effector memory cells that secrete IL-4 and IL-13.[38] Dupilumab has been used to treat CTCL associated with pruritus.[39] However, use of dupilumab has been associated with worse outcomes in CTCL as its antagonistic effect at the primary IL-13 receptor increases serum IL-13 levels. Elevated IL-13 levels result in increased binding to IL-13α2, creating a paracrine loop that drives Th2-mediated pathogenesis.[40]

In addition to skewing CD4 helper T cells to their Th2 phenotype, proposed mechanisms for the association between AD and CTCL include immunosurveillance, drug toxicity side effects, and chronic inflammation by the immune system.[41] A meta-analysis of five cohort studies and 18 case-control studies suggests that AD has an increased association with CTCL (RR = 1.43).[34] It was noted that some of the cases likely began as CTCL, but were misdiagnosed as AD.

In Sweden and Denmark, a cohort study found that adults with AD treated with topical corticosteroids had 10% higher incidence rate (3 vs 0.3) of CTCL than patients with AD that were untreated. Furthermore, when comparing the use of tacrolimus to corticosteroids for AD treatment, adults had approximately 3 times higher incidence rate (9.5 vs 3.1) of developing CTLC. One potential confounder is that patients with less severe AD were less likely to require treatment.[42] These findings underscore the positive association of AD with CTCL, emphasizing the crucial role of accurate diagnosis for each condition. It is essential to differentiate between the two, as treatments intended for AD may inadvertently worsen the prognosis of CTCL. The introduction of dupilumab as a recent second-line treatment option for moderate-to-severe AD adds another layer of complexity, given its negative impacts on the prognosis of CTCL. These observations highlight the need for further research to better understand the interplay between AD treatments and the development and progression of CTCL.

OTHER MALIGNANCIES
Breast cancer

There seems to be a positive correlation between breast cancer (BC) and AD. In a review by Sadeghi and Shirkhoda, researchers reviewed literatures regarding the associations between AD and BC. Ultimately, it was found that there seems to be an increased risk for BC in patients with a general history of allergies, but more specifically with allergic conditions, such as AD and allergic rhinitis. All but one study in the review showed a statistically significant increase in risk of BC in those previously diagnosed with AD.[43] However, studies that reported the significant risk of BC were likely influenced by confounders, such as age, parity, breast feeding, and other gynecologic histories. In Taiwan, of 18749 women with AD according to the National Health Insurance (NHI) Research Database, the SIR of breast cancer was 1.2.[22]

In a retrospective cohort study by Hedderson and colleagues, a population of patients diagnosed with moderate (requiring topical therapy or photo-therapy treatment) or severe (requiring systemic treatment) AD were analyzed for incidence of ma-lignancies. Though both men and women were included in the study, evaluation for BC was con-ducted for only women. The incidence ratio (IR) for breast cancer in those with AD was significantly high [IR for moderate AD = 2.2 (95% CI 1.6–3.0); IR for severe AD = 0.5 (95% CI 0.1–3.9)]. It is pro-posed that the chronic inflammation and altered cell-mediated immunity in AD may play a role in increased tumorigenesis, resulting in higher IRs for breast cancer.[44] Of note, while this study included a large population of women (n = 4542), all participants were located in Northern California, which limits its generalisability. Additionally there was no control group with which to compare pa-tients with and without AD.

Lung cancer

The association between AD and lung cancer was investigated in a study involving 756 patients diag-nosed with lung cancer in Quebec, revealing an in-verse association with malignancy (OR = 0.34). This study also looked at asthma's association with lung cancer, although it did not specify how many patients with AD also had asthma. To help mitigate recall errors in patients, the OR was also calculated from patients who reported receiving treatment for AD. With this more stringent defini-tion of AD, there was a further decrease in associ-ation, yet the difference between AD and AD treated with medication was not statistically signif-icant (OR = 0.29).[19]

Similarly, in Taiwan, a survey of the NHI, which covers over 95% of their population, found AD to be associated with a decreased risk of lung cancer (SIR = 0.76). Interestingly, this study looked at diagnosis of both asthma and AD, as approxi-mately 25% of patients with AD also had asthma. In relation to 18 cancers analyzed, the combination further reduced the association with malignancy (SIR = 0.73) compared to AD alone (SIR = 0.97).[22]

However, a study conducted in England using the primary health care data from the Clinical Prac-tice Research Datalink GOLD and the National Pa-tient Registry in Denmark found an increased

hazard ratio (HR = 1.08) for AD with lung cancer af-ter adjusting for confounders.[5] This study did not assess the prevalence of asthma among patients with AD.

The close clinical association of AD with asthma may also influence its association with lung can-cer. It is important for analyses of AD and lung can-cer to account for additional risk factors, such as cigarette smoke exposure and occupational exposure.

Glioma

There has generally been found to be an inverse association between AD and glioma risk.[45–47] The majority of studies investigating this associa-tion have shown AD, and potentially other atopic conditions, may be protective against glioma. An investigation by Pouchieu and colleagues utilized the data from the CERENAT study (CEREbral tu-mors: a NATional study) to further examine allergy patient history and glioma risk.[47] Other atopic con-ditions, such as allergic rhinitis and asthma, were considered. There was a significant negative cor-relation between allergy and glioma (OR = 0.52, 95% CI 0.36–0.75) with increased allergic condi-tions further reducing glioma risk (p-trend = 0.001). The protective effect of allergy on glioma was greater in women.[47] Greater exploration into the mechanism behind these associations may yield further understanding.

Additional studies affirmed this relationship by looking at incidental glioma cases with sibling, friend, and clinic-based controls.[48] A history of allergic conditions was obtained, which ultimately revealed an inverse association with glioma that was also dose-dependent on the number of atopic conditions. AD specifically demonstrated the in-verse association with only the friend control group (OR = 0.42, 95% CI 0.15–1.18). Having multiple control groups to compare with the glioma-diagnosed patients is a strength of this study. A Mendelian randomisation study by Disney-Hogg and colleges produced very similar results with an OR of 0.96 (95% CI 0.93–1.00, P = .041) be-tween AD and glioma. This relationship could possibly be due to the fact that the immunosup-pression characteristic of glioma suppresses the development and presentation of atopic dis-eases.[45] A report from 2016 also supported the fact that history of allergy reduces glioma risk, but suggested that it is respiratory allergy specifically that provides the protective role. The data from other studies suggest that it may be elevated IgE levels that help to protect against glioma.[46]

While most literature shows the negative associ-ation between AD and glioma, not all studies found similar results. Lupatsch and colleagues looked for associations between childhood brain tumors (CBT), including glioma, and factors like day care attendance, early childhood infections, childhood contact with animals, in addition to a history of atopy. While farm and pet contacts were shown to be inversely associated with CBTs, no association was found with any allergy conditions. These findings could be due to recall or selection bias, considering the retrospective nature of the study.[49]

SUMMARY

In this review, the authors describe the association of AD with various skin malignancies, solid tumors, and hematologic malignancies. We focused on the evolving therapies for AD, hypothesizing the mechanism by which new pharmacological interventions may impact the association of AD with various malignancies. AD, although primarily characterized by skin manifestations, is part of a broad inflammatory response that affects the entire body and is many times described as presenting as an atopic triad with asthma and allergies.[50] While the authors' review focuses solely on AD association with malignancies, it is important to consider the correlation of asthma with AD in lung cancers.

In terms of skin cancer association with AD patients, it appears that there is an increased risk of BCC and SCC. One potential confounder is that patients with AD are more likely to be seen by dermatologists, and this confounder seems to be present for the association of AD with CTCL. However, this association may be due to similarities in biology, especially in melanoma, where C6A6 appears to be expressed in both AD and melanoma. Subtle differences in integrins highlight the different roles the immune system plays in AD and melanoma. Melanoma is enriched for integrin β8, which activates TGFβ, a key immunosuppressive cytokine that dampens antigen presentation by dendritic cells and prevents T cell activation. On the contrary, integrin β6 has increased expression in AD due to proinflammatory cytokines TNF-α and IL-1β.[7]

Several studies on the association of cancers of the gastrointestinal (GI) tract with AD were published recently.[18,20,21] Inflammatory response of the skin may extend to the GI tract.[50] A recent meta-analysis focusing on all allergic conditions indicates inverse association with CRC and mortality from CRC.[51] In particular, the key cytokine IL-13 appears to play a role in both the pathogenesis in AD and an improved prognosis in CRC.[52] The introduction of new AD treatments targeting IL-13 raises questions about how their blockade may impact the negative association of AD with CRC.

Stratifying for risk factors for GI tract malignancies may shed light on the association with AD. Helicobacter pylori——a risk factor for gastric and esophageal cancer—— is less prevalent in developed countries.[53] Interestingly, the association of AD and H. pylori was studied with a lack of an overall general consensus being reached.[54] The authors also consider that esophageal cancer has different rates across the world along with varying prevalence of SCC and adenocarcinoma.[25] CRC is also preventable with colonoscopy as removal of precancerous lesions in patients may skew results of association with AD.[55] The authors also recognize that diet is a major player in the development of many GI cancers.[56,57] Most of the research on association of GI cancers and AD focused on the Americas, Europe, and East Asia. Whether differences in the association can be credited to diet, immune system, or exposure to different allergens still remains a question. Studying this association in other parts of the world may lend some insight.

There seems to be an increased association between AD and hematologic malignancies. CTCL is of particular interest due to it often being confused with AD due to similar presentations.[37] CTCL has an increased association with AD and of growing concern is that treatments for AD may increase the severity of CTCL.[40] This emphasizes that, even with their similar presentations, subtle differences in their mechanism and biology can cause exacerbation of CTCL with treatments targeting IL-13. It will be interesting to monitor drug development for AD and see if the authors can find treatments that work for both AD and CTCL given the diagnostic challenges.

The trends between GI cancers and hematologic malignancies suggest that increased immune surveillance from immune activation may account for decreased incidence of GI malignancies. However, this may correlate with an increased association with various hematologic malignancies, as constant stimulation of the immune system may lead to accumulation of hematopoietic stem cells with uncontrolled replication potential.[58]

CLINICS CARE POINTS

- AD is frequently associated with other allergic conditions, which may also play a role in its association with certain cancers such as in the lung.

- Understanding cancer predisposition patients have due to AD may aid in more proactive preventative care for these individuals.

- TCIs, a second-line treatment for AD, despite their black box warning for immunosuppressive effects, are not associated with increased risk of melanoma.

- Overlap between commonly used treatments, such as glucocorticoids for both AD and ALL, may be an important factor for the inverse association risk between these two conditions.

- CTCL is often misdiagnosed as AD, and an accurate diagnosis of both is important for treatment. This is especially important before IL4/ IL13 blockade.

- New biologic drugs targeting specific molecular pathways may influence the association of AD with malignancies, which should be explored by further research.

- Understanding how these therapies influence cancer risk may better guide providers in treatment decision-making.

- While certain trends appeared on the association of AD with specific cancers, it is hard to draw definite conclusions, and considering genetic, environmental, and other risk factors on a case-to-case basis is still needed.

DISCLOSURE

No funding was secured for this study.

REFERENCES

1. Savva M, Papadopoulos NG, Gregoriou S, et al. Recent advancements in the atopic dermatitis mechanism. Front Biosci (Landmark Ed) 2024; 29(2):84.
2. Kim J, Kim BE, Leung DYM. Pathophysiology of atopic dermatitis: clinical implications. Allergy Asthma Proc 2019;40(2):84–92.
3. Cipolat S, Hoste E, Natsuga K, et al. Epidermal barrier defects link atopic dermatitis with altered skin cancer susceptibility. Elife 2014;3:e01888. Fuchs E, ed.
4. Anand P, Kunnumakara AB, Sundaram C, et al. Cancer is a preventable disease that requires major lifestyle changes. Pharm Res 2008;25(9):2097–116.
5. Mansfield KE, Schmidt SAJ, Darvalics B, et al. Association between atopic eczema and cancer in England and Denmark. JAMA Dermatol 2020;156(10): 1086–97.
6. Holm Nielsen S, Port H, Møller Hausgaard C, et al. A fragment of type VI collagen alpha-6 chain is elevated in serum from patients with atopic dermatitis, psoriasis, hidradenitis suppurativa, systemic lupus erythematosus and melanoma. Sci Rep 2023;13(1): 3056.
7. Nguyen BA, Ho J, De La Cruz Diaz JS, et al. TGFβ activating integrins β6 and β8 are dysregulated in inflammatory skin disease and cutaneous melanoma. J Dermatol Sci 2022;106(1):2–11.
8. Gandini S, Stanganelli I, Palli D, et al. Atopic dermatitis, naevi count and skin cancer risk: a meta-analysis. J Dermatol Sci 2016;84(2):137–43.
9. Lam M, Zhu JW, Tadrous M, et al. Association between topical calcineurin inhibitor use and risk of cancer, including lymphoma, keratinocyte carcinoma, and melanoma: a systematic review and meta-analysis. JAMA Dermatol 2021;157(5): 549–58.
10. Dyer RK, Weinstock MA, Cohen TS, et al. Predictors of basal cell carcinoma in high-risk patients in the VATTC (VA Topical Tretinoin Chemoprevention) trial. J Invest Dermatol 2012;132(11):2544–51.
11. Jensen AO, Svaerke C, Körmendiné Farkas D, et al. Atopic dermatitis and risk of skin cancer: a Danish nationwide cohort study (1977-2006). Am J Clin Dermatol 2012;13(1):29–36.
12. Gamba CA, Tang JY. Does a history of eczema predict a future basal cell carcinoma? J Invest Dermatol 2012;132(11):2497–9.
13. Cho JM, Davis DMR, Wetter DA, et al. Association between atopic dermatitis and squamous cell carcinoma: a case-control study. Int J Dermatol 2018; 57(3):313–6.
14. Hagströmer L, Ye W, Nyrén O, et al. Incidence of cancer among patients with atopic dermatitis. Arch Dermatol 2005;141(9):1123–7.
15. Olesen AB, Engholm G, Storm HH, et al. The risk of cancer among patients previously hospitalized for atopic dermatitis. J Invest Dermatol 2005;125(3):445–9.
16. Zhu Y, Wang H, He J, et al. Atopic dermatitis and skin cancer risk: a systematic review. Dermatol Ther 2022;12(5):1167–79.
17. Prizment AE, Folsom AR, Cerhan JR, et al. History of allergy and reduced incidence of colorectal cancer, Iowa Women's Health Study. Cancer Epidemiol Biomarkers Prev 2007;16(11):2357–62.
18. Choi YJ, Han K, Jin EH, et al. Allergic diseases and risk of malignancy of gastrointestinal cancers. Cancers 2023;15(12):3219.
19. El-Zein M, Parent ME, Kâ K, et al. History of asthma or eczema and cancer risk among men: a population-based case-control study in Montreal, Quebec, Canada. Ann Allergy Asthma Immunol 2010;104(5): 378–84.
20. Zhan ZQ, Huang ZM, Zeng RQ, et al. Association between atopic dermatitis and colorectal cancer: tet2 as a shared gene signature and prognostic biomarker. J Cancer 2024;15(5):1414–28.
21. Chou WY, Lai PY, Hu JM, et al. Association between atopic dermatitis and colorectal cancer risk: a

nationwide cohort study. Medicine (Baltim) 2020; 99(1):e18530.

22. Hwang CY, Chen YJ, Lin MW, et al. Cancer risk in patients with allergic rhinitis, asthma and atopic dermatitis: a nationwide cohort study in Taiwan. Int J Cancer 2012;130(5):1160–7.

23. Meng C, Sun L, Shi J, et al. Exploring causal correlations between circulating levels of cytokines and colorectal cancer risk: A Mendelian randomization analysis. Int J Cancer 2024. https://doi.org/10.1002/ijc.34891.

24. Grille VJ, Campbell S, Gibbs JF, Bauer TL. Esophageal cancer: the rise of adenocarcinoma over squamous cell carcinoma in the Asian belt. J Gastrointest Oncol 2021;12(Suppl 2):S339–49.

25. Liu Y, Gu Y, Zhou J, et al. Mendelian randomization analysis of atopic dermatitis and esophageal cancer in East Asian and European populations. World Allergy Organ J 2024;17(2):100868.

26. Li J, Wang W, Wang K, et al. Interleukin 13 participates in terminal differentiation of esophageal squamous cell carcinoma cells. J Gastrointest Oncol 2022;13(4):1571–8.

27. Liang Z, Liu J, Jin H, et al. Potential correlation between eczema and hematological malignancies risk: a systematic review and meta-analysis. Front Med 2022;9:912136.

28. Mohamed MEF, Bhatnagar S, Parmentier JM, et al. Upadacitinib: mechanism of action, clinical, and translational science. Clin Transl Sci 2024;17(1):e13688.

29. Iznardo H, Roé E, Serra-Baldrich E, et al. Efficacy and Safety of JAK1 Inhibitor Abrocitinib in Atopic Dermatitis. Pharmaceutics 2023;15(2):385.

30. Fleischmann R, Mysler E, Bessette L, et al. Long-term safety and efficacy of upadacitinib or adalimumab in patients with rheumatoid arthritis: results through 3 years from the SELECT-COMPARE study. RMD Open 2022;8(1):e002012.

31. Hu Q, Bian Q, Rong D, et al. JAK/STAT pathway: Extracellular signals, diseases, immunity, and therapeutic regimens. Front Bioeng Biotechnol 2023;11.

32. Degryse S, Cools J. JAK kinase inhibitors for the treatment of acute lymphoblastic leukemia. J Hematol Oncol 2015;8:91.

33. CLINICAL TRIAL/NCT03571321- UChicago Medicine. Available at: https://www.uchicagomedicine.org/find-a-clinical-trial/clinical-trial/irb171110. Accessed July 2, 2024.

34. Legendre L, Barnetche T, Mazereeuw-Hautier J, et al. Risk of lymphoma in patients with atopic dermatitis and the role of topical treatment: A systematic review and meta-analysis. J Am Acad Dermatol 2015;72(6):992–1002.

35. Natoli A, Lüpertz R, Merz C, et al. Targeting the IL-4/IL-13 signaling pathway sensitizes Hodgkin lymphoma cells to chemotherapeutic drugs. Int J Cancer 2013;133(8):1945–54.

36. Holtick U, Vockerodt M, Pinkert D, et al. STAT3 is essential for Hodgkin lymphoma cell proliferation and is a target of tyrphostin AG17 which confers sensitization for apoptosis. Leukemia 2005;19(6):936–44.

37. Hinkamp CA, Gupta S, Keshvani N. Severe adult-onset atopic dermatitis mistaken for cutaneous T-cell lymphoma in a medically complex patient. BMJ Case Rep 2020;13(3):e234445.

38. Mazzetto R, Miceli P, Tartaglia J, et al. Role of IL-4 and IL-13 in Cutaneous T Cell Lymphoma. Life 2024;14(2):245.

39. Talmon A, Elias S, Rubin L, et al. Dupilumab for cancer-associated refractory pruritus. J Allergy Clin Immunol Glob 2023;2(3):100128.

40. Park A, Wong L, Lang A, et al. Cutaneous T-cell lymphoma following dupilumab use: a systematic review. Int J Dermatol 2023;62(7):862–76.

41. Josephs DH, Spicer JF, Corrigan CJ, et al. Epidemiological associations of allergy, IgE and cancer. Clin Exp Allergy 2013;43(10):1110–23.

42. Castellsague J, Kuiper JG, Pottegård A, et al. A cohort study on the risk of lymphoma and skin cancer in users of topical tacrolimus, pimecrolimus, and corticosteroids (Joint European Longitudinal Lymphoma and Skin Cancer Evaluation - JOELLE study). Clin Epidemiol 2018;10:299–310.

43. Sadeghi F, Shirkhoda M. Allergy-related diseases and risk of breast xancer: the role of skewed immune system on this association. Allergy Rhinol (Providence) 2019;10:2152656719860820.

44. Hedderson MM, Asgari MM, Xu F, et al. Rates of malignancies among patients with moderate to severe atopic dermatitis: a retrospective cohort study. BMJ Open 2023;13(3):e071172.

45. Disney-Hogg L, Cornish AJ, Sud A, et al. Impact of atopy on risk of glioma: a Mendelian randomisation study. BMC Med 2018;16(1):42.

46. Amirian ES, Zhou R, Wrensch MR, et al. Approaching a scientific consensus on the association between allergies and glioma risk: a report from the glioma international case-control study. Cancer Epidemiol Biomarkers Prev 2016;25(2):282–90.

47. Pouchieu C, Raherison C, Piel C, et al. Allergic conditions and risk of glioma and meningioma in the CERENAT case-control study. J Neuro Oncol 2018;138:271–81.

48. Il'yasova D, McCarthy B, Marcello J, et al. Association between glioma and history of allergies, asthma, and eczema: a case-control study with three groups of controls. Cancer Epidemiol Biomarkers Prev 2009;18(4):1232–8.

49. Lupatsch JE, Bailey HD, Lacour B, et al. Childhood brain tumours, early infections and immune stimulation: A pooled analysis of the ESCALE and ESTELLE

case-control studies (SFCE, France). Cancer Epidemiol 2018;52:1–9.

50. Darlenski R, Kazandjieva J, Hristakieva E, et al. Atopic dermatitis as a systemic disease. Clin Dermatol 2014;32(3):409–13.

51. Ma W, Yang J, Li P, et al. Association between allergic conditions and colorectal cancer risk/mortality: a meta-analysis of prospective studies. Sci Rep 2017;7(1):5589.

52. Formentini A, Braun P, Fricke H, et al. Expression of interleukin-4 and interleukin-13 and their receptors in colorectal cancer. Int J Colorectal Dis 2012; 27(10):1369–76.

53. Salih BA. Helicobacter pylori infection in developing countries: the burden for how long? Saudi J Gastroenterol 2009;15(3):201–7.

54. Zuel-Fakkar NM, Girgis SA. Study of Helicobacter pylori in children with atopic dermatitis. J Egyptian Women's Dermatologic Society 2011;8(1):17.

55. Bretthauer M, Løberg M, Wieszczy P, et al. Effect of colonoscopy screening on risks of colorectal cancer and related death. N Engl J Med 2022;387(17): 1547–56.

56. Karagulle M, Fidan E, Kavgaci H, et al. The effects of environmental and dietary factors on the development of gastric cancer. J BUON 2014;19(4):1076–82.

57. Song M, Garrett WS, Chan AT. Nutrients, foods, and colorectal cancer prevention. Gastroenterology 2015; 148(6):1244–60.e16.

58. Craver BM, El Alaoui K, Scherber RM, Fleischman AG. The critical role of inflammation in the pathogenesis and progression of myeloid malignancies. Cancers 2018;10(4):104.

Atopic Dermatitis
The Role of the Social Determinants of Health on Severity and Access to Care

Nanette B. Silverberg, MD

KEYWORDS

• Atopic dermatitis • Social determinants • Comorbidities • Poverty • Medicaid • Black • Hispanic

KEY POINTS

• Atopic dermatitis (AD) is noted to be more severe in Black and Hispanic children.
• Patients with AD having more limited resources may have difficulty treating the disease.
• Access to therapeutics and medical care for AD in underserved populations is frought with barriers including prior authorizations, step edits, and drug formulary exclusions.

INTRODUCTION

Atopic dermatitis (AD) is a multi-system inflammatory disease with skin manifestations beginning for most patients in the first 12 months of life.[1] The disease is manifested by red, oozing skin lesions in typical locations,[2] causing many comorbidities including infectious, atopic, and psychiatric.[3] One-half of children persist in having disease after age 8 years,[1] and half of these children will persist with risk factors including hand eczema, allergic rhinitis, and early onset.[4] The estimated adult prevalence of AD in the United States is currently 7.3%, although this may be an underestimate.[5] Childhood estimates of AD are 12.97% in the United States, although some studies suggest numbers as high as 17.1%.[6,7]

SOCIAL DETERMINANTS OF AD

AD disproportionately affects Black and Hispanic individuals in the United States in numbers and severity. This is *not* explained by genetics for African American adults, highlighting the role of the social determinants of health.[8] Environmental and social factors are prominently associated with AD severity and health care determinants, for all Skin of Color populations including Black and Asian populations,[9] but also for all children living below the poverty level. Ultimately children are highly susceptible to risk factors for childhood AD ranging.

The severity of AD includes less prescribing of specific commonly used therapeutics,[9] as well as difficulty accessing therapies for individuals on Medicaid and Children's Health Insurance Program (CHIP). Barriers to access include lack of inclusion of common medications on formulary, frequent and cumbersome prior authorizations, and difficulty in finding available formularies online, limiting patient engagement.[9–12] "Black and Hispanic children are less likely to see providers, have more severe disease, more persistent disease, greater school absenteeism, and more likely to need multiple visits for good disease control."[13] Other associations include increased emergency department (ED) usage, less access to dermatology and allergy, and more comorbidities of asthma and allergy which reduce quality of life.[13] Allergic disease in general is associated with paternal education, rent, food insecurity, and food stamps.[14]

The mnemonic GLUM has been used to summarize social determinants in AD: garbage in the streets, lack of community support/lower educational level of parents, under the poverty line, and Medicaid/single mothers.[13] There are no prospective regional data on the life course of patients with AD, comparing individuals of different

Department of Dermatology, Icahn School of Medicine at Mt Sinai, 5 East 98th Street, 5th Floor, New York, NY 10029, USA
E-mail address: Nanette.silverberg@mountsinai.org

Dermatol Clin 42 (2024) 635–638
https://doi.org/10.1016/j.det.2024.06.003
0733-8635/24/© 2024 Elsevier Inc. All rights are reserved, including those for text and data mining, AI training, and similar technologies.

races, and ethnicities, from infancy through adulthood addressing social determinants as they occur alongside disease. Zip codes have not been explored in relationship to AD. Geospatial localization is quite limited in urban cities that are not completely segregated, such as New York City, where public housing projects can be built adjacent to high-rent properties.

The socially at-risk populations in the United States may include a large segment of the population because all the commonly recognized social determinants of health[15]: Insurance—Medicaid and CHIP,[13] Race/ethnicity—Black and Hispanic (this is not mutually exclusive from Medicaid and CHIP given the higher percentage of Black and Hispanic children/adults on public health insurance), Asian children, and children of immigrants,[13] socioeconomic status—single parent households/living under the poverty level,[13] Education—lower level of parental education[13]/poor health literacy,[16] relationship status—single-mother households,[13] rural or urban—rural has reduced access to care due to transportation, urban has more garbage[13] and poor air quality,[17] employment—missed work-days,[18] income—living under the poverty level,[13] and language—readability is limited for online "educational tools".[13,19]

One disparity in AD is the difficulty in characterizing AD based erythema in children of color. It is not known what percentage of children fail prior authorizations based on the difficulty of observance of the AD features on clinical examination. In this setting education is extremely important—for physicians and parents, and readablity of documents at a 6th grade level is needed to improve education on AD care. Additionally, erythema-free or color-neutral scoring is needed for prior authorizations in order to level the eligibility for therapeutic intervention with Caucasians[20]

Another way to look at AD is through an expanded socie-ecological model of health care depicted in **Fig. 1**, based on a modification of the model by Purnell.[21,22]

In greater detail, the model is as follows: Level 1: Individual Factors: Genetic Factors and Psychological Factors, which can be targeted for early intervention. Filaggrin mutations are uncommon in Black patients, but may be more common in Asian children. Level 2: Family/Friends and Social Support help parents and families cope with the difficulties of AD on the household including time consumption, cost, and office visits. Level 3: Cultural Groups, Religious Networks, and Internet Networks—Church groups have been poorly explored for interventions, but represent an untapped resource. Studies show that patients and caregivers receive their information (or more likely

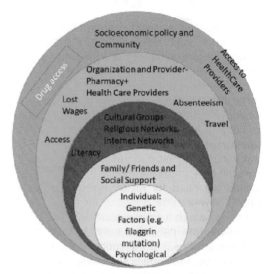

Fig. 1. A socioeconomic model of atopic dermatitis.

misinformation) from online resources, although many Web sites are difficult to read.[22] Level 4: Organization and Provider Level includes issues such as access, prescribing, communication, prior authorization, man power, physician burnout, and language barriers. Level 5: Socioeconomic policy and community highlights the vagaries of poverty as they affect daily life and long-term opportunity in patients and families of children with AD. Altered opportunity includes less ability to take on jobs, avoidance of careers with associated wetwork, and opportunity lost associated with missed work. Although there is overlap between organization and provider, there are differences in the role of policy in access to health care providers (HCP) and pharmacists, including formularies relevant to AD care, step-edits, and pharmacy benefit managers, among the barriers that policy creates in the United States.

Social factors that have been linked to AD include lack of social support, as noted in single mothers, and living in dirty environments with garbage in the streets.[13] Furthermore, AD is socially isolating and stigmatizing, reducing the patient and caregiver's ability to form relationships. Social stigmatization and poor attachment have also been linked to AD.[22] An example might be a mother of a child with AD who is concerned about leaving her child with a babysitter given the difficulty of the child's skin care.[23]

Economic factors play a strong role in the socioeconomic model of AD, with financial factors including living below the poverty level[13] and participation in Medicaid/CHIP health insurance.[13] Black patients, in particular, are at greater risk of the burden of financial impact of AD, with notable harmful financial impact in the setting of being Black with Medicaid.[22]

Environmental factors affecting AD include an urban environment with increased pollution and comorbid asthma as well as a rural environment with reduced physical proximity to dermatologic care. Other environmental factors include the presence of garbage in the streets, mold, pests, and poor air circulation, the latter 3 are linked to AD and asthma in Mexican immigrants.[24]

Healthcare policy is a concerning aspect of AD care. First and foremost the cost of emollients in the United States has skyrocketed during the COVID-19 pandemic, creating a rapid increase in strain on families living in poverty with a child with AD. In the United States only 3 states cover bland emollients on their Medicaid/CHIP formularies,[11] and there is a tremendous need for simple interventions to be covered.[25] Because topical bland emollients are the first intervention in AD in all guidelines, it is exceedingly problematic that they are not provided for free to the underpriveleged seeking public assistance health care for their child with AD and for adults as well. Poor access to topical agents has been a focus of multiple publications that address social disparity in AD.[6,11,23] The cost of emollients for AD is $35.13 to $316.75, and this can be crippling for the impoverished patient and family.[26] Ultimately, the financial feasibility of access to petrolatum or paraffin-based emollients, through universal emollient access for Medicaid and CHIP patients without prescription, may be a mechanism of early-intervention that ultimately prevents. In particular, there is evidence to demonstrate that not covering the cost of AD care for individuals in poverty causes significant social harm to the family.[27] Other policies include limited access to standard-of-care topical corticosteroids.[11] The usage of extensive prior authorization steps adds a minimum of 3 weeks of delay before a medication is received.[28] Health care factors that are associated with AD include comorbid asthma, and food allergies, which negatively impact quality of life in AD.[29,30]

SUMMARY

In order to develop potential intervention strategies in the future, the problem of AD disparity has to be better defined. As a result, further research is needed, and specifically in the form of trials of interventional programs. Interventional programs are vital, as there are populations that benefit from emollient-prevention and other that do not. Practical functional availability of emollients and topical therapeutics may ease financial strain. Other opportunities may exist in community-based care.

Increasing education with regards to the appearance of disease and color-neutral scoring systems are needed. Improving readability of handouts and online documents by translating into multiple languages at a sixth grade reading level is needed to reduce literacy barriers.

CLINICS CARE POINTS

- The disease course of patients with Atopic Dermatitis is negativly impacted by social determinants of health.
- Social determinants implicated in disease activity include race and ethnicity, as well as public assistance.
- Care of the atopic dermatitis patient requires consideration of all of the levels of social determinant factors in order to produce the best outcomes.

DISCLOSURE

N.B. Silverberg has been an advisor or received honoraria from Amryt, Incyte, Lilly, Regeneron/Sanofi, and Verrica Pharmaceuticals. There was no funding obtained for this work.

REFERENCES

1. Kay J, Gawkrodger DJ, Mortimer MJ, et al. The prevalence of childhood atopic eczema in a general population. J Am Acad Dermatol 1994;30(1):35–9.
2. Eichenfield LF, Tom WL, Chamlin SL, et al. Guidelines of care for the management of atopic dermatitis: section 1. Diagnosis and assessment of atopic dermatitis. J Am Acad Dermatol 2014;70(2):338–51.
3. Davis DMR, Drucker AM, Alikhan A, et al. American Academy of Dermatology Guidelines: Awareness of comorbidities associated with atopic dermatitis in adults. J Am Acad Dermatol 2022;86(6):1335–6.e18.
4. Mortz CG, Andersen KE, Dellgren C, et al. Atopic dermatitis from adolescence to adulthood in the TOACS cohort: prevalence, persistence and comorbidities. Allergy 2015;70(7):836–45.
5. Chiesa Fuxench ZC, Block JK, Boguniewicz M, et al. Atopic dermatitis in america study: a cross-sectional study examining the prevalence and disease burden of atopic dermatitis in the US adult population. J Invest Dermatol 2019;139(3):583–90.
6. Silverberg JI, Simpson EL. Associations of childhood eczema severity: a US population-based study. Dermatitis 2014;25(3):107–14.
7. Hanifin JM, Reed ML, Eczema Prevalence and Impact Working Group. A population-based survey

of eczema prevalence in the United States. Dermatitis 2007;18(2):82–91.

8. Abuabara K, You Y, Margolis DJ, et al. Genetic ancestry does not explain increased atopic dermatitis susceptibility or worse disease control among African American subjects in 2 large US cohorts. J Allergy Clin Immunol 2020;145(1):192–8.e11.

9. Marcelletti A, Shan DM, Abdi W, et al. Special considerations of atopic dermatitis in skin of color. Adv Exp Med Biol 2024;1447:45–57. PMID: 38724783.

10. Bell MA, Whang KA, Thomas J, et al. Racial and ethnic disparities in access to emerging and front-line therapies in common dermatological conditions: a cross-sectional study. J Natl Med Assoc 2020; 112(6):650–3. Epub 2020 Jul 5. PMID: 32641259.

11. Kamara M, Kuo AM, Stein SL, et al, PeDRA Skin of Color Special Interest Group. Disparities in availability of skin therapies found in public assistance formularies. J Am Acad Dermatol 2022;87(2):411–7.

12. Loiselle AR, Thibau IJ, Johnson JK, et al. Financial and treatment access burden associated with atopic dermatitis comorbidities. Ann Allergy Asthma Immunol 2024;132(2):243–5.

13. Kuo A, Silverberg N, Fernandez Faith E, et al. A systematic scoping review of racial, ethnic, and socioeconomic health disparities in pediatric dermatology. Pediatr Dermatol 2021;38(Suppl 2):6–12.

14. Federman A, Wisnivesky JP. Unveiling the reasons for disparities in prevalence of asthma and allergic conditions in Black children: The role of socioeconomic status. J Allergy Clin Immunol 2024;153(4): 983–4. Epub 2024 Feb 3. PMID: 38316270.

15. Purnell TS, Calhoun EA, Golden SH, et al. Achieving health equity: closing the gaps in health care disparities, interventions, and research. Health Aff (Millwood) 2016;35(8):1410–5.

16. Leeman EJ, Loman L. Health literacy in adult patients with atopic dermatitis: A cross-sectional study. J Allergy Clin Immunol Glob 2024;3(2):100218.

17. Ai S, Liu L, Xue Y, et al. Prenatal exposure to air pollutants associated with allergic diseases in children: which pollutant, when exposure, and what disease? a systematic review and meta-analysis. Clin Rev Allergy Immunol 2024;19. https://doi.org/10.1007/s12016-024-08987-3.

18. Kemp AS. Cost of illness of atopic dermatitis in children: a societal perspective. Pharmacoeconomics 2003;21(2):105–13.

19. Skrzypczak T, Skrzypczak A, Szepietowski JC. Readability of patient electronic materials for atopic dermatitis in 23 languages: analysis and implications for dermatologists. Dermatol Ther (Heidelb) 2024;14(3):671–84. Epub 2024 Feb 24.

20. Mitchell KN, Tay YK, Heath CR, et al. Review article: Emerging issues in pediatric skin of color, Part 2. Pediatr Dermatol 2021;38(Suppl 2):30–6. Epub 2021 Oct 27. PMID: 34708446.

21. https://www.cdc.gov/violenceprevention/about/social-ecologicalmodel.html. [Accessed 17 April 2024].

22. Purnell TS, Calhoun EA, Golden SH, et al. Achieving health equity: closing the gaps in health care disparities, interventions, and research. Health Aff (Millwood) 2016; 35(8):1410–5.

23. Mueller SM, Hongler VNS, Jungo P, et al. Fiction, falsehoods, and few facts: cross-sectional study on the content-related quality of atopic eczema-related videos on YouTube. J Med Internet Res 2020;22(4): e15599.

24. Afshari M, Kolackova M, Rosecka M, et al. Unraveling the skin; a comprehensive review of atopic dermatitis, current understanding, and approaches. Front Immunol 2024;15:1361005.

25. Chovatiya R, Begolka WS, Thibau IJ, et al. Financial burden and impact of atopic dermatitis out-of-pocket healthcare expenses among black individuals in the United States. Arch Dermatol Res 2022; 314(8):739–47.

26. Scollan ME, Garzon MC, Lauren CT. State medicaid coverage of over-the-counter moisturizers: A cost-effective management strategy for atopic dermatitis? Pediatr Dermatol 2022;39(5):838–45. Epub 2022 Aug 12. PMID: 35960142.

27. Diao L, Allshouse A, Diaz-Castillo S, et al. Housing environments and child health conditions among recent Mexican immigrant families: a population-based study. J Immigr Minor Health 2010;12(5):617–25.

28. Scollan ME, Garzon MC, Lauren CT. State medicaid coverage of over-the-counter moisturizers: A cost-effective management strategy for atopic dermatitis? Pediatr Dermatol 2022;39(5):838–45.

29. Hecht B, Frye C, Holland W, et al. Analysis of prior authorization success and timeliness at a community-based specialty care pharmacy. J Am Pharm Assoc 2003;61(4S):S173–7.

30. Weidinger S, Simpson EL, Silverberg JI, et al. Burden of atopic dermatitis in pediatric patients: an international cross-sectional study. Br J Dermatol 2023;4:ljad449.

UNITED STATES POSTAL SERVICE®

Statement of Ownership, Management, and Circulation (All Periodicals Publications Except Requester Publications)

1. Publication Title DERMATOLOGIC CLINICS	**2. Publication Number** 000 – 705	**3. Filing Date** 9/18/2024
4. Issue Frequency JAN, APR, JUL, OCT	**5. Number of Issues Published Annually** 4	**6. Annual Subscription Price** $447.00

7. Complete Mailing Address of Known Office of Publication (Not printer) (Street, city, county, state, and ZIP+4®)

ELSEVIER INC.
230 Park Avenue, Suite 800
New York, NY 10169

Contact Person
Malathi Samayan
Telephone (Include area code)
91-44-4299-4507

8. Complete Mailing Address of Headquarters or General Business Office of Publisher (Not printer)

ELSEVIER INC.
230 Park Avenue, Suite 800
New York, NY 10169

9. Full Names and Complete Mailing Addresses of Publisher, Editor, and Managing Editor (Do not leave blank)

Publisher (Name and complete mailing address)

Dolores Meloni, ELSEVIER INC.
1600 JOHN F KENNEDY BLVD. SUITE 1600
PHILADELPHIA, PA 19103-2899

Editor (Name and complete mailing address)

Stacy Eastman, ELSEVIER INC.
1600 JOHN F KENNEDY BLVD. SUITE 1600
PHILADELPHIA, PA 19103-2899

Managing Editor (Name and complete mailing address)

PATRICK MANLEY, ELSEVIER INC.
1600 JOHN F KENNEDY BLVD. SUITE 1600
PHILADELPHIA, PA 19103-2899

10. Owner (Do not leave blank. If the publication is owned by a corporation, give the name and address of the corporation immediately followed by the names and addresses of all stockholders owning or holding 1 percent or more of the total amount of stock. If not owned by a corporation, give the names and addresses of the individual owners. If owned by a partnership or other unincorporated firm, give its name and address as well as those of each individual owner. If the publication is published by a nonprofit organization, give its name and address.)

Full Name	Complete Mailing Address
WHOLLY OWNED SUBSIDIARY OF REED/ELSEVIER, US HOLDINGS	1600 JOHN F KENNEDY BLVD. SUITE 1600 PHILADELPHIA, PA 19103-2899

11. Known Bondholders, Mortgagees, and Other Security Holders Owning or Holding 1 Percent or More of Total Amount of Bonds, Mortgages, or Other Securities. If none, check box. ▶ ☐ None

Full Name	Complete Mailing Address
N/A	

12. Tax Status (For completion by nonprofit organizations authorized to mail at nonprofit rates) (Check one)
The purpose, function, and nonprofit status of this organization and the exempt status for federal income tax purposes:
☒ Has Not Changed During Preceding 12 Months
☐ Has Changed During Preceding 12 Months (Publisher must submit explanation of change with this statement)

PS Form **3526**, July 2014 [Page 1 of 4 (see instructions page 4)] PSN: 7530-01-000-9931   PRIVACY NOTICE: See our privacy policy on www.usps.com.

---

13. Publication Title DERMATOLOGIC CLINICS		**14. Issue Date for Circulation Data Below** JULY 2024	

15. Extent and Nature of Circulation		**Average No. Copies Each Issue During Preceding 12 Months**	**No. Copies of Single Issue Published Nearest to Filing Date**
a. Total Number of Copies (Net press run)		115	130
b. Paid Circulation (By Mail and Outside the Mail)	(1) Mailed Outside-County Paid Subscriptions Stated on PS Form 3541 (Include paid distribution above nominal rate, advertiser's proof copies, and exchange copies)	62	85
	(2) Mailed In-County Paid Subscriptions Stated on PS Form 3541 (Include paid distribution above nominal rate, advertiser's proof copies, and exchange copies)	0	0
	(3) Paid Distribution Outside the Mails Including Sales Through Dealers and Carriers, Street Vendors, Counter Sales, and Other Paid Distribution Outside USPS®	42	32
	(4) Paid Distribution by Other Classes of Mail Through the USPS (e.g., First-Class Mail®)	5	6
c. Total Paid Distribution (Sum of 15b (1), (2), (3) and (4)) ▶		108	123
d. Free or Nominal Rate Distribution (By Mail and Outside the Mail)	(1) Free or Nominal Rate Outside-County Copies included on PS Form 3541	6	6
	(2) Free or Nominal Rate In-County Copies Included on PS Form 3541	0	0
	(3) Free or Nominal Rate Copies Mailed at Other Classes Through the USPS (e.g., First-Class Mail)	0	0
	(4) Free or Nominal Rate Distribution Outside the Mail (Carriers or other means)	1	1
e. Total Free or Nominal Rate Distribution (Sum of 15d (1), (2), (3) and (4)) ▶		7	7
f. Total Distribution (Sum of 15c and 15e) ▶		115	130
g. Copies not Distributed (See Instructions to Publishers #4 (page #3)) ▶		0	0
h. Total (Sum of 15f and g) ▶		115	130
i. Percent Paid (15c divided by 15f times 100)		93.91%	94.62%

* If you are claiming electronic copies, go to line 16 on page 3. If you are not claiming electronic copies, skip to line 17 on page 3.

PS Form **3526**, July 2014 (Page 2 of 4)

16. Electronic Copy Circulation	**Average No. Copies Each Issue During Preceding 12 Months**	**No. Copies of Single Issue Published Nearest to Filing Date**
a. Paid Electronic Copies ▶		
b. Total Paid Print Copies (Line 15c) + Paid Electronic Copies (Line 16a) ▶		
c. Total Print Distribution (Line 15f) + Paid Electronic Copies (Line 16a) ▶		
d. Percent Paid (Both Print & Electronic Copies) (16b divided by 16c × 100) ▶		

☒ I certify that 50% of all my distributed copies (electronic and print) are paid above a nominal price.

17. Publication of Statement of Ownership

☒ If the publication is a general publication, publication of this statement is required. Will be printed in the OCTOBER 2024 issue of this publication.   ☐ Publication not required.

18. Signature and Title of Editor, Publisher, Business Manager, or Owner

Malathi Samayan   Date 9/18/2024

Malathi Samayan - Distribution Controller

I certify that all information furnished on this form is true and complete. I understand that anyone who furnishes false or misleading information on this form or who omits material or information requested on the form may be subject to criminal sanctions (including fines and imprisonment) and/or civil sanctions (including civil penalties).

PS Form **3526**, July 2014 (Page 3 of 4)   PRIVACY NOTICE: See our privacy policy on www.usps.com

Moving?

Make sure your subscription moves with you!

To notify us of your new address, find your **Clinics Account Number** (located on your mailing label above your name), and contact customer service at:

Email: **journalscustomerservice-usa@elsevier.com**

800-654-2452 (subscribers in the U.S. & Canada)
314-447-8871 (subscribers outside of the U.S. & Canada)

Fax number: **314-447-8029**

Elsevier Health Sciences Division
Subscription Customer Service
3251 Riverport Lane
Maryland Heights, MO 63043

ELSEVIER